Road Map to a Healthy Eating Lifestyle

How to Reach Your Weight Goals and Keep the Weight Off

Mark Simpson, Ph.D.

AI Text Disclosure and Image Credits: Portions of the text were developed with assistance from OpenAI's ChatGPT; the author reviewed, revised, and takes responsibility for the final manuscript. Some images were created using OpenAI's ChatGPT image-generation tools; remaining images are original to the author or separately credited.

Cover Design by Mark Simpson

Printed in the United States of America First Printing, 2026

First Edition

ISBN 978-1-933306-04-9 (Hardback)
ISBN 978-1-933306-05-6 (Paperback)
ISBN 978-1-933306-06-3 (Digital)

Published by EDCOT® Press
A registered trademark

Dedication

To all who embark on the journey toward a healthy eating lifestyle

Acknowledgments

I am deeply grateful for the encouragement, care, and support I have received from so many individuals and groups as I embark on this journey. I especially want to note my sincere appreciation to:

- My Water's Edge Church family and friends in Henderson, Kentucky.
- My friends and colleagues across the country and around the world.
- The stylists at Shear Madness in Newburgh, Indiana.
- The baristas at the Grimm Road Starbucks in Newburgh, Indiana.
- The doctors and medical personnel at Evansville Primary Care, Indiana.

Above all, I give thanks to the Lord for His daily provisions, grace, and the strength He provides to remain faithful and consistent on this journey. His guidance and sustaining presence are acknowledged with humility and gratitude.

Table of Contents

Chapter 1: Road Map to a Healthy Eating Lifestyle

A Practical Guide to Sustainable Healthy Eating

"If the LORD delights in a man's way, He makes his steps firm." – Psalm 37:23 (NIV)

Imagine waking up tomorrow knowing exactly what to eat, when to eat, and how each meal moves you closer to your objectives. The *Road Map to a Healthy Eating Lifestyle* will help you arrive, making each choice easier, leading to real, observable results from everyday achievements—yours and mine.

To make these ideas more practical, the *Road Map* uses the journey metaphor. This approach frames your experience clearly. For example, weight loss appears as miles traveled, and changes in body size become distance markers. These metaphors offer simple, visual cues to recognize progress and relate daily efforts to your long-term goals.

Because practicality guides this *Road Map,* it is written in everyday language. You are the driver on this journey, and the aim is to help you make informed choices without relying on complex or technical explanations. While some medical or nutritional terms are necessary, they are introduced carefully and explained to support your understanding without overwhelming you with jargon.

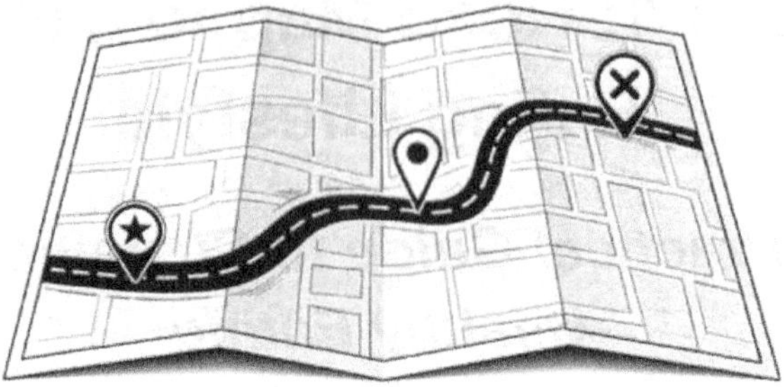

Along your journey, you may encounter well-meaning people who question or doubt your progress. These comments often come from individuals used to seeing you at a different stage of health and may mistake your positive changes, especially your appearance, as unhealthy. Measure your progress by your own goals and your body's response—not by external opinions. *The clearest signals come from your body and your primary care physician.*

Your Personal Destination

The information in this *Road Map* aims to provide you with a step-by-step guide that helps you set up your own destination and understand along the way:

- What may be happening in your body
- What changes are most likely to improve your health
- What experiences you may have on your own journey

This *Road Map* is grounded in authentic experiences, practical insights, and behavioral patterns commonly encountered during the transition to healthier eating habits. Because some of these approaches may not have been successful for you in previous attempts at weight loss, please try them again. Several of the principles followed in this *Road Map* involve modifications to traditional keto-based approaches, carb addiction recovery principles, carnivore-centered nutrition, fasting protocols, and time-restricted eating strategies. In many ways, the *Road Map* reflects more of a ketovore approach that melds all of these together to achieve healthy eating.

1. **Road Map to a Healthy Eating Lifestyle** – Practical Principles for Lasting Change.
   Chapter 1 (this chapter) introduces you to the journey ahead by establishing the *Road Map* metaphor that frames the entire book. It shows how the chapters work together, helping you to understand how to use the *Road Map* as your guide to a healthy eating lifestyle.

2. **Guidelines for Personal Success (GPS)** – Understanding the Route Ahead of You
   Chapter 2 establishes a shared language for the journey. It functions as a legend for the *Road Map,* defining foundational concepts while introducing GPS not as satellite navigation, but as Guidelines for Personal Success. By clarifying expectations and core ideas at the outset, Chapter 2 prepares you to apply the operational principles and practices that follow in subsequent chapters.

3. **Eating Healthy** – Observing the Rules of the Road
   Chapter 3 outlines the essential operating principles for daily eating. It explains the importance of allowing your body time each morning before the first meal, introduces structured eating windows such as one or two meals per day, and presents fasting as a supportive framework that builds on the body's natural rhythms rather than as an extreme practice. Intermittent fasting and alternate day fasting are described as tools that reinforce healthy eating patterns and improve metabolic flexibility. Chapter 3 emphasizes prioritizing protein to support metabolic health

and muscle preservation, and pairing healthy fats intentionally with protein to support fullness and steady energy. It also emphasizes the careful, selective use of supplements as supportive aids rather than primary drivers of progress. Throughout, an emphasis on food quality, structure, and thoughtful decision-making reinforces the rules that help you maintain steady, predictable, and sustainable progress.

4. **Foods to Eat** – Knowing the Approved Lanes
   Chapter 4 identifies foods that support forward movement on your journey. Emphasis is placed on organically produced, properly sourced, and responsibly raised foods, including grass-fed and free-range options. Natural sweeteners that minimize metabolic disruption are highlighted, along with stable, minimally processed fats such as cold-pressed extra virgin olive oil, coconut oil, MCT oil, and avocado oil. Full-fat dairy options, when tolerated, are presented as supportive rather than something you need to fear.

5. **Foods to Avoid** – Avoiding the Closed Roads
   Chapter 5 identifies foods that consistently derail progress. Highly processed products, conventionally farm-raised options, industrial seed oils, and foods heavily based on corn and soy are presented as closed roads—paths that may appear convenient but ultimately lead you away from metabolic health and long-term success.

6. **Staying on Course** – Rest Stops, Side Roads, and Ongoing Maintenance

   Chapter 6 brings together the practical realities that impact forward momentum with healthy eating. It addresses expected and unexpected delays such as eating while traveling, holiday meals, dining invitations, and other changes in daily eating patterns. Sleep and appropriate physical activity are also addressed as essential components that help keep the body refreshed and strong for the journey. Finally, monitoring overall progress is suggested and can be as simple as keeping track of changes in body weight and clothing sizes rather than using complex tracking methods. Collectively, these strategies emphasize that lasting success depends not on avoiding interruptions, but on responding wisely and pressing on with the journey.

7. **Starting Your Journey** – Entering the On-Ramp
   Chapter 7 provides a structured and practical way to begin following the *Road Map to a Healthy Eating Lifestyle.* Organized as a week-by-week progression of the principles and practices of healthy eating, it focuses on establishing food quality selection first, then gradually introduces eating windows, intermittent fasting, and varying eating patterns to reduce metabolic predictability. The emphasis is on adaptability rather than rigidity, encouraging you to build sustainable habits.

8. **Enjoying the Destination** – Maintaining Your Success
   Chapter 8 shifts the focus from reaching the destination to living there. It emphasizes enjoyment, consistency, and long-term stewardship of the progress you have achieved, reinforcing that this *Road Map* is not about temporary change, but about sustaining a healthy eating lifestyle over time.

9. **Roadside Assistance** – Consulting Reliable Resources.
   Chapter 9 is the closing section, designed as a place you can return to over time to continue exploring reliable, up-to-date information on healthy eating. The resources listed here provide ongoing insight, clarification, and reinforcement of the principles presented throughout this *Road Map*. As your understanding grows and new questions emerge, this section serves as a reliable

reference, offering trusted resources that help you stay informed while continuing to live a healthy eating lifestyle.

10. **Traveler's Checklist** – Essentials for a Healthy Eating Lifestyle
    Chapter 10 brings together the essential food choices and guiding principles of the *Road Map to a Healthy Eating Lifestyle,* which are further detailed in the other chapters. It is intended as a reference point, not a stand-alone guide, and assumes the understanding developed along the journey rather than replacing it.

When Previous Attempts Fell Short of the Destination

It is understandable to approach a new eating plan with skepticism if you have tried similar approaches before without lasting success. Many people have experimented with keto, carnivore, low-carbohydrate eating, fasting, or other structured plans, only to regain weight or feel that the approach was unsustainable. Over time, those experiences can shape expectations and lead to the belief that "this *Road Map* will not work for me," regardless of the reasons similar (but not identical) eating plans may have fallen short in the past.

This *Road Map* asks you to consider a different starting point. Rather than treating healthy eating as a short-term intervention or a rigid set of rules, the *Road Map* is grounded more in metabolic principles that explain *why* certain principles and practices work and how the body adapts to changes in eating patterns over time. Past attempts may have failed you not because you lacked discipline or commitment, but because the approach was incomplete, overly restrictive, or disconnected from how your metabolism functions. By focusing on understanding the metabolic impact of the foods you eat rather than just seeking quick results, this *Road Map* can help you move forward with a clearer sense of direction and long-term success, even if previous routes that on the surface appeared similar did not lead where you hoped.

When GLP-1 Medications Are Part of the Journey

For those using GLP-1 medications—such as Ozempic, Wegovy, Mounjaro, Zepbound, or similar—this *Road Map* provides guidance that supports what these medications cannot do on their own: teach discernment, reinforce intentional nourishment, and establish sustainable eating patterns. While these medications may assist with appetite regulation and short-term weight loss, they do not by themselves create the habits or metabolic understanding needed for long-term success. In this way, the *Road Map* serves as an essential companion, helping translate temporary medical support into lasting lifestyle change that can be sustained well beyond the period of medication use.

Initial Key Terminology

As you encounter various healthy eating resources, you may encounter several medical terms. The last section of the *Road Map* provides a map-like legend of several key terms, defined in simpler terms, to help you understand these resources. The definitions provided are not intended to be technical or exhaustive. Instead, they provide practical explanations that will help orient you as new ideas are introduced and revisited across the chapters. Some terms may feel familiar, others may be new, and a few may take on more depth of meaning as your understanding of healthy eating unfolds. When that happens, the terminology "legend" can be revisited as needed to confirm direction and understanding.

The terminology list is not exhaustive, and all the terms are important. But here are a handful of terms it is helpful to know upfront.

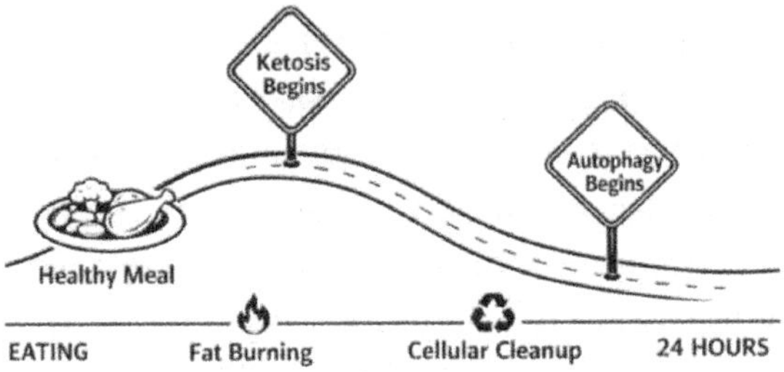

Autophagy – a natural cellular recycling process activated during fasting, in which damaged or dysfunctional cells are broken down and reused for repair and renewal.

Cortisol – a hormone produced by the adrenal glands that plays a central role in the body's stress response, energy regulation, and blood sugar balance. Cortisol levels naturally follow a daily rhythm, rising in the morning and tapering throughout the day. Chronic stress, inadequate sleep, or metabolic strain can disrupt this rhythm, potentially affecting appetite, fat storage, and overall progress in a healthy eating lifestyle.

Ghrelin – a hormone produced primarily in the stomach that signals hunger to the brain; levels typically rise before meals and fall after eating. During dietary changes, especially reduced carbohydrate intake or fasting, this hormone signaling may temporarily increase as the body adjusts to new eating patterns.

Ketosis – a metabolic state in which the body primarily burns fat for fuel and produces ketones as an energy source due to low carbohydrate intake.

Mitochondria – the structures within your cells responsible for producing energy. They convert the food you eat into usable fuel that powers movement, bodily functions, and overall metabolic activity. Because cells respond directly to the components found in food, not just calorie counts or marketing claims, the quality and processing of what you eat can either support or disrupt mitochondrial function. Foods that appear healthy on the surface may still interfere with this process at the cellular level. When mitochondria are well supported, energy production is steady and efficient; when they are disrupted, fatigue and stalled metabolic progress can occur even when calorie intake seems appropriate.

Processed Foods – foods altered from their natural state through industrial processing, often containing refined sugars, seed oils, and additives that disrupt metabolic health.

Seed Oils – industrially processed vegetable oils high in omega-6 fatty acids. Excessive consumption is commonly associated with inflammation and metabolic disruption.

Subcutaneous Fat – fat stored just beneath the skin. It is the type of fat most visible on the body and is commonly associated with appearance and body shape. While subcutaneous fat contributes to overall body weight, it is generally less metabolically active than visceral fat and is often reduced later in the healthy eating journey.

Visceral Fat – fat stored deep within the abdominal cavity, surrounding internal organs such as the liver, pancreas, and intestines. This type of fat is metabolically active and closely associated with insulin resistance, inflammation, and increased risk of chronic disease. Reducing visceral fat is a primary health goal of this *Road Map*, as improvements in metabolic health often begin internally before visible changes occur.

IMPORTANT DISCLAIMER: *Road Map to a Healthy Eating Lifestyle* is not medical advice and is provided solely for general informational purposes. The concepts described are not intended to diagnose, treat, cure, or prevent any medical condition. Any information contained in this work should be discussed with one's primary care physician, and medical guidance should be sought before beginning, altering, or discontinuing any eating, fasting, activity, or lifestyle practice. Each reader's circumstances, health status, and needs differ, and the decision to follow any principle presented in this work rests solely with the reader. Neither the author nor the publisher assumes responsibility for any outcomes, concerns, or complications resulting from the use of any information contained in this work, whether in whole or in part. Discontinue any practice immediately if you feel unwell or uncomfortable.

Key Points to Remember from Chapter 1

The following key points from Chapter 1 serve as road signs to guide your progress on your healthy eating lifestyle journey.

- The *Road Map* is designed to guide your development and maintenance of a healthy eating lifestyle.
- Rely on your GPS—Guidelines for Personal Success—to stay oriented.
- Understanding your starting point through honest observation rather than a judgmental perspective is essential.

- Principles set the direction for your healthy eating, while practices are more flexible and should be aligned with your personal health needs and conditions.
- Progress depends on intentional nourishment, not eating less.
- Treat this *Road Map* as a guide you return to, especially when it is time to adjust your eating plan.

May your journey begin successfully, and you reach your destination safely!

Chapter 2: Guidelines for Personal Success (GPS)

Understanding the Route Ahead of You

"Trust in the LORD with all your heart and lean not on your own understanding; in all your ways acknowledge him, and he will make your paths straight." – Proverbs 3:5-6 (NIV)

Today, most of us taking a road trip will use an online map to chart our route. These maps utilize GPS, a satellite-based Global Positioning System that provides precise information about your location, direction, speed, and time anywhere on Earth. GPS works by receiving signals from a network of satellites and calculating position based on the time it takes those signals to reach a receiver. Similarly, the *Road Map* has its own GPS—Guidelines for Personal Success—that assist you along your healthy eating journey. Location, direction, speed, and time with this GPS can best be thought of as follows:

- **Location** – your current eating patterns, habits, and metabolic state, providing an honest assessment of where you are starting and where you are positioned at any given moment.
- **Direction** – the intentional food choices, fasting practices, and lifestyle decisions that orient you toward improved metabolic health and sustained progress.
- **Speed** – the pace at which results unfold, influenced by consistency, adherence to principles, and the body's natural adaptation processes.

- **Time** – the long-term commitment required to establish, reinforce, and maintain a healthy eating lifestyle rather than seeking short-term outcomes.

While GPS-based maps have replaced traditional paper maps still available in many gas stations and rest stops, both share a common feature: a legend that explains the meanings of the symbols on the map. With paper maps, the legend is usually found in a rectangular box. The legend on GPS-based maps is dynamic, revealing different symbols and levels of detail as the map is magnified or reduced, allowing the traveler to see what is most relevant at each stage of the journey. Chapter 8 includes this map-like legend of terms you will likely encounter on your journey.

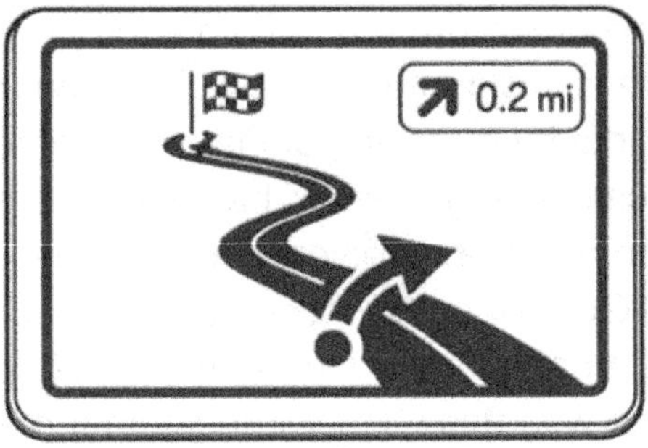

Understanding Your Starting Point

Understanding your starting point is an essential part of any journey. Before directions can be followed or progress measured, you must know where you are beginning. This *Road Map* does not assume a single entry point, because no two eating journeys start from the same place.

Your own starting point includes your current eating patterns, your relationship with food, your energy levels, and how your body responds to what you eat and when you eat. Some readers may already be limiting carbohydrates, others may be eating frequently throughout the day, and many may fall somewhere in between. None of these positions disqualifies you from the journey. They simply describe your present location.

Identifying your hunger signals, meal timing, food choices, and how you feel after eating provides valuable information for your healthy eating journey. Awareness creates clarity, and clarity makes direction meaningful. Without it, changes become guesswork rather than intentional movement.

Understanding your starting point also means recognizing that progress is personal. Comparing your journey to someone else's can distort expectations and lead to frustration. The *Road Map* is designed to guide your movement forward, not to measure you against another traveler's pace or path.

As you continue following the *Road Map*, your Guidelines for Personal Success GPS will necessarily need to be updated to your "healthy eating location" over time, just as a Global Positioning System GPS recalculates as you walk or travel in a vehicle. Understanding the importance of periodically checking your GPS allows you to adjust your direction, pace, and expectations as your body adapts and your understanding of healthy eating deepens.

Principles Versus Practices

Principles keep you oriented and provide a sense of direction. Practices are the daily actions that carry you toward living out those principles. Throughout this *Road Map*, principles function as the underlying road signs that shape decision-making, while practices are the practical ways those principles are lived out day by day.

Principles are stable. They do not change with your circumstances, preferences, or seasons of life. They help you evaluate choices, adjust when needed, and remain oriented even when specific strategies shift. *Practices, by contrast, are flexible.* They reflect how principles are applied at a particular time, based on your current needs, context, and level of readiness.

For example, a principle may emphasize reducing insulin exposure or prioritizing whole, nourishing foods. The practice that expresses that principle might involve changing meal timing, adjusting your food selections, or experimenting with different eating windows. As your body adapts and your understanding grows, the practices may change, but the principle remains constant.

This distinction between principles and practices matters because lasting change is rarely sustained through rigid routines alone. When practices are followed without understanding the principles behind them, frustration often follows when results slow or circumstances change. When principles are understood first, practices can be adjusted thoughtfully rather than abandoned altogether.

Throughout this *Road Map,* you will encounter various eating approaches, fasting patterns, and lifestyle recommendations. These are presented as practices—tools that serve the principles, not rules that define success or failure. You are encouraged to engage them intentionally, observing how your body responds, and adjust your healthy eating journey as needed.

By learning to think in terms of principles and practices, you gain the confidence to navigate your journey. Rather than asking whether you are following a plan perfectly, you can ask whether your current practices align with the principles that support long-term metabolic health. This mindset allows progress to continue even as conditions change.

As you move forward, keep this distinction in view: principles set the direction; practices move you toward the destination.

Together, they allow the *Road Map* to remain both structured and adaptable as you continue developing a healthy eating lifestyle.

It is important to note that one principle that applies across every stage of this *Road Map* is the importance of eating adequately, not merely eating less. As eating patterns change and fasting is introduced, sufficient protein intake serves as a safeguard to preserve lean mass and support the body's ongoing needs. While specific protein targets and food choices will be addressed later, the principle remains consistent: progress is supported when nourishment is intentional rather than restrictive.

How to Follow this *Road Map*

This *Road Map* is designed to guide you, not to rush you. You should not expect to master every concept all at once or apply every practice immediately. Just as with any journey, understanding the route comes before traveling it, and forward movement happens one decision at a time.

Each of the following chapters in the *Road Map to a Healthy Eating Lifestyle* builds upon the previous chapters, though the *Road Map* is not strictly linear. You may find yourself moving forward, revisiting earlier chapters or sections, or pausing to reflect on your understanding of your personal healthy eating journey. This flexibility is intentional. Progress is best measured not by speed, but by consistency and direction over time.

As you follow this *Road Map*, pay attention to how your body responds, how your energy changes, and how your relationship with food changes over time. Adjustments are part of the journey, and are not signs of failure. When challenges arise, use them as opportunities to recalibrate rather than reasons to abandon the route. This is especially important to remember when side roads appear along your journey, such as eating less-than-healthy foods during the holidays, unhealthy foods at special events, or occasional treats. *Side roads will happen,* and learning how those side roads impact your healthy eating journey can help you get back on track and stay on track even when you encounter them.

The *Road Map* does not ask you to compare your progress to others or to meet external benchmarks. It invites you instead to stay attentive to your own signals and to make informed choices that align with your long-term health goals. This goal is not about perfection, but rather is about stewardship—learning to care for your body with intention, patience, and compassion.

As you move into the following chapters, keep the guiding concepts from this first chapter in view. Use this healthy eating GPS to stay oriented, return to the legend when needed, and remember that every person's journey is different.

Updating Your Journey

As with any journey, it is helpful to have a place for you to return to for guidance, updates, and support along the way. Throughout *Road Map to a Healthy Eating Lifestyle,* various resources, tools, and references are mentioned to assist you as you continue developing a healthy eating lifestyle. Just as roadways can be modified over time, the following link serves as a central reference point where you can find resources mentioned in the chapters, along with additional materials and ongoing updates. This online resource is designed to remain current and responsive, allowing the *Road Map* to continue serving you beyond the pages of this book.

https://edcot.info/healthy-eating

Key Points to Remember from Chapter 2

The following key points from Chapter 2 serve as road signs to guide your progress on your healthy eating lifestyle journey.

- Use the *Road Map* metaphor to guide your healthy eating journey with clarity and purpose.
- Rely on GPS—Guidelines for Personal Success—to stay oriented in direction, pace, and expectations.
- Refer to the Key Terms Legend in the "Road Assistance" chapter of the *Road Map* to ensure consistent understanding throughout the journey.
- Begin by understanding your starting point through honest observation rather than judgment.
- Let stable principles guide your decisions while allowing practices to remain flexible.
- Prioritize intentional nourishment, including adequate protein intake, rather than focusing solely on eating less.
- Measure progress through patience, consistency, and compassion rather than perfection.
- Follow the *Road Map* as a guide you return to and adjust over time.
- Use the https://edcot.info/healthy-eating weblink to access referenced materials and ongoing updates.

Chapter 3: Eating Healthy

Observing the Rules of the Road

"If you find honey, eat just enough—too much of it, and you will vomit." – Proverbs 25:16 (NIV)

Having established the overall *Road Map* and its guiding framework in Chapter 1, Chapter 3 focuses on how healthy eating can be practiced day by day. The emphasis here is not on perfection and hard-and-fast rule-following, but on learning and consistently applying a set of practical guidelines that keep progress steady, predictable, and sustainable.

Just as roadways function best when drivers understand and follow established rules, healthy eating guidelines improve your results when clear boundaries govern timing, structure, and the choices you make. These guidelines reduce confusion, limit unnecessary detours, and help your body respond more efficiently to nourishment. Rather than relying on constant decision-making or willpower, Chapter 2 emphasized concepts that simplify your daily eating and support long-term change.

The operational principles in Chapter 3 address when eating occurs, how your meals are structured, and why specific patterns support better outcomes than others. Topics such as delayed morning eating, fasting, meal composition, macronutrient balance, and food quality are presented as coordinated practices rather than isolated techniques. When applied together, they create a unified approach that supports your healthy eating as a lifestyle rather than as a temporary intervention.

Please Note: As your healthy eating journey progresses, it is vitally important that you are getting enough protein to support your metabolic health. As you become accustomed to eating less—and desiring to eat less—you will be tempted not to eat enough or even at all. To prevent muscle loss rather than fat loss, be sure to eat enough protein on your eating days. The rule of thumb is to eat one gram of protein for every pound of your goal weight.

Understanding How Fat Loss Occurs

Before you begin applying the timing, fasting, and meal structuring principles, it is helpful to understand how your body typically responds to these changes. Fat loss does not occur uniformly, and progress is often internal before it becomes visible. This *Road Map* is intentionally designed to improve metabolic health first, which means it usually targets visceral fat before subcutaneous fat.

Visceral fat, which surrounds your internal organs, is more metabolically active and more responsive to changes in insulin levels. Practices such as delayed eating, intermittent fasting, and alternate day fasting reduce insulin stimulation and allow your body to access stored energy more readily. As insulin levels remain lower for more extended periods, visceral fat is often mobilized first, leading to improvements in energy, appetite regulation, and overall metabolic health—even as outward appearance changes more slowly.

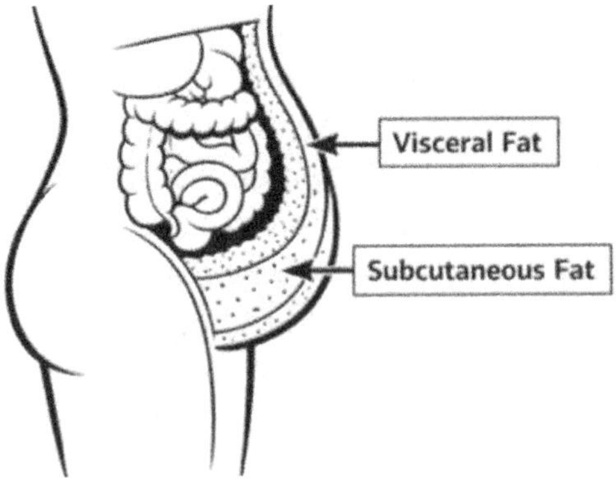

Subcutaneous fat, which lies just beneath your skin, is typically more resistant and is often reduced later in the journey. Because this type of fat is less metabolically active, visible changes such as movement on the scale or changes in body shape may lag behind internal improvements. Understanding this sequence helps prevent discouragement and reinforces the importance of measuring progress by health outcomes rather than appearance alone.

Protein prioritization plays a critical role during this process. As visceral fat is mobilized, adequate protein intake helps protect lean muscle mass and supports metabolic stability. Without sufficient protein, your body may lose muscle alongside fat, slowing progress and undermining long-term health. By pairing fasting strategies with protein-centered meals, this *Road Map* supports fat loss while preserving strength and function.

This approach differs from many calorie-focused eating plans that emphasize immediate weight loss without regard for fat type or muscle preservation. By prioritizing metabolic health, this *Road Map* emphasizes sustainable progress. Internal changes lay the groundwork for visible results, and over time, reductions in subcutaneous fat typically follow the metabolic improvements already underway.

As visceral fat is reduced, you will often notice improvements that go well beyond changes on the scale. Energy levels may increase, mental clarity may improve, appetite may become calmer, and movement may feel easier as pressure on internal organs decreases. Over time, these internal changes translate into visible physical differences, such as improvements in your posture, breathing, and overall body composition, rather than changes limited to belly fat alone. Unlike calorie-restricted diets that may produce early weight loss while leaving metabolic health unchanged or muscle mass diminished, this *Road Map* improves metabolic health and fat loss together. As you continue to progress, your body increasingly reflects these more profound changes through healthier composition, more effortless movement, and better overall physical function.

Misconceptions About Weight Loss

After researching the advice of various health advisors and medical practitioners throughout my journey, I became aware of misconceptions about weight loss. Traditional food plans, dieting principles, and eating practices have changed over the years. What was once common advice is now being challenged as the focus on healthy eating shifts to what happens inside the body at the cellular level rather than what you see on the outside.

Many people expect their bodies to respond quickly once food choices change. When that does not happen, it is easy to assume something is wrong or that the approach is not working. But your body's ability to shift between carbohydrate and fat as fuel develops gradually. Early hunger, uneven energy, or difficulty extending time between meals often reflect how accustomed the body is to frequent carbohydrate intake rather than a lack of progress.

Metabolic Flexibility Spectrum

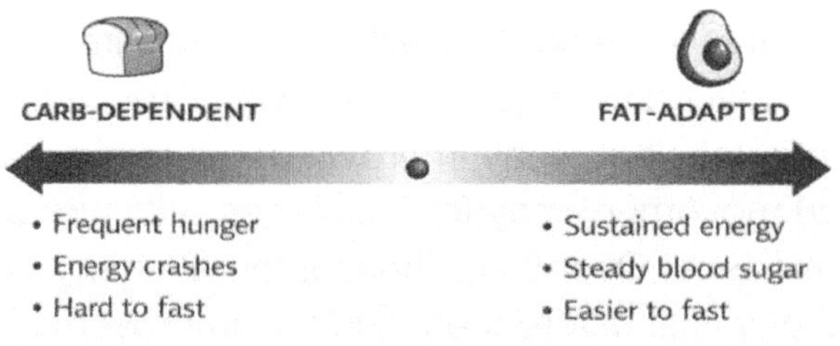

Here are some additional assumptions and examples of what happens in practice to illustrate the changes you undergo when adopting a healthy eating lifestyle.

Assumption: You must join a gym to lose weight.
In Practice: Exercise supports muscle and overall health, but weight loss is primarily driven by metabolic regulation and eating patterns rather than by gym attendance.

Assumption: You must eat less total food to lose weight.
In Practice: Eating until comfortably full using real, nutrient-dense foods supports satisfaction and reduces the urge to snack or abandon the plan.

Assumption: You must buy supplements, protein shakes, bars, or powders to succeed.
In Practice: Supplements may offer limited support, but consistent food quality and eating habits matter far more.

Assumption: If you stop eating carbohydrates, weight loss and health improvements will happen immediately.
In Practice: Reducing carbohydrates supports metabolic healing, but progress unfolds over time as the body adapts.

Assumption: You must exercise intensely or frequently for weight loss to work.
In Practice: Gentle, consistent movement preserves muscle and supports metabolism without requiring strenuous workouts.

Assumption: Feeling hungry means the plan is working.
In Practice: Persistent hunger signals an unsustainable approach and often leads to overeating or abandoning the plan.

Assumption: Weight loss should happen quickly if the method is correct.
In Practice: Gradual change is more reliable and reflects lasting metabolic improvement rather than short-term fluctuation.

Assumption: Daily changes on the scale determine success or failure.
In Practice: Weight naturally fluctuates due to hydration, digestion, and stress, making trends more meaningful than daily numbers.

Assumption: If weight loss slows or pauses, something is broken.
In Practice: Plateaus are common during metabolic healing and often reflect normal adaptation rather than failure.

Assumption: Low-carbohydrate eating means small portions.
In Practice: Satisfying meals built around protein and healthy fats are essential for appetite control and consistency.

Assumption: Skipping meals randomly is the same as fasting.
In Practice: Structured fasting works best when intentional and paired with adequate nutrition.

Assumption: More restriction always produces better results.
In Practice: Excessive restriction raises stress hormones and cravings, often undermining progress.

Assumption: Supplements can compensate for poor food choices.
In Practice: No supplement can replace consistent, high-quality eating habits.

Assumption: Weight loss is mainly about willpower.
In Practice: Sustainable progress depends on structure, preparation, and metabolic stability rather than constant self-control.

Setting Eating Times

Establishing consistent eating times is one of the foundational rules of the road for healthy eating. Within this *Road Map,* timing functions as an organizing framework rather than a restrictive rule set. Clear boundaries around when your eating begins and ends each day reduce metabolic confusion, minimize impulsive decisions, and support steady, sustainable progress.

Begin your day with a deliberate pause before your first meal. Waiting approximately 90 minutes after waking allows the body to complete its natural morning transition, including hormone regulation and metabolic activation, without immediately shifting into digestion. This delay helps limit early insulin stimulation, allowing the liver to complete its morning metabolic transition and signaling the body to move gradually from energy release to digestion, thereby supporting metabolic flexibility. It is essential to establish a consistent eating window(s) to help you control your eating habits—whether it is one window (OMAD) or two windows for two meals per day (TMAD). By doing so, you help your body learn when nourishment is available and when it is not.

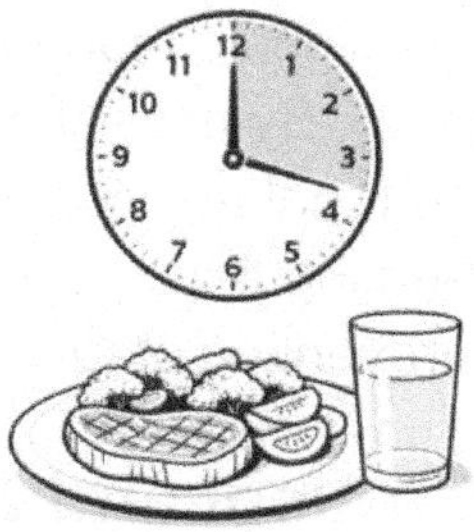

When your meal timing and eating patterns remain identical day after day, your body may adapt by becoming more efficient rather than continuing to release stored energy, which can lead to diminishing returns. To counter this effect, you can introduce occasional, intentional variations within established boundaries so that your progress does not stall. These may include modestly extending the fasting window, alternating between one and two meals a day, or slightly shifting meal timing from time to time. These adjustments are strategic rather than reactive and help you preserve metabolic responsiveness without abandoning structure.

Establishing a clear end-of-eating time each day is also an essential part of maintaining a healthy eating structure. When you eat late into the evening, insulin activity is extended into hours better suited for rest and repair. Defining when eating stops supports circadian alignment and can improve sleep quality, which, in turn, influences appetite regulation the following day. During fasting periods, you can use water, black coffee, or green tea to support your fast without undermining its success.

Structured eating times help retrain behavior. When eating windows are clearly defined, it becomes easier for you to distinguish true physiological hunger from eating driven by stress, boredom, or emotional cues—a crucial distinction if you are recovering from carbohydrate dependence. Eating within set times functions like traffic signals and guardrails, helping you evaluate your hunger signals thoughtfully rather than just obeying them automatically. By not eating for 90 minutes after you wake up, defining your eating windows, and establishing your end-of-day end-of-eating times, you keep your eating progress steady while preventing stagnation and fatigue.

Understanding Cortisol and Eating Windows

It is essential to understand how stress and stress hormones can influence eating patterns, even when food choices and routines are well established. Cortisol, often referred to as the body's primary stress hormone, plays a normal and necessary role in regulating energy availability, blood sugar, and the body's response to physical and emotional demands.

When cortisol levels remain elevated for extended periods due to chronic stress, inadequate sleep, or persistent schedule disruption, it can subtly influence appetite and food preferences. Elevated cortisol tends to increase hunger signals, promote cravings for quick energy sources, and encourage fat storage, particularly when combined with frequent carbohydrate intake. Over time, this can make maintaining established eating patterns feel more difficult, even when effort and intention remain unchanged.

Consuming protein as the first meal of the day supports the body's transition from the overnight fast without amplifying stress-related hormonal responses. Introducing protein instead of carbs provides your body with the amino acids that support muscle preservation and tissue maintenance without provoking a sharp rise in blood glucose or insulin. This allows cortisol levels to follow their normal downward course rather than being further stimulated by a rapid influx of carbohydrates.

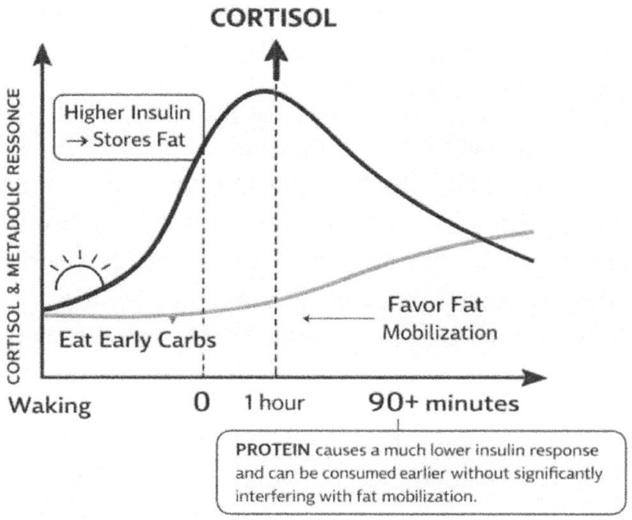

Protein intake also supports the continuation of beneficial metabolic processes initiated during sleep. Overnight, the body engages in repair, renewal, and hormonal regulation. Beginning the day with protein helps preserve these effects by stabilizing blood sugar, moderating appetite signals, and reducing the likelihood of reactive hunger later in the day. In contrast to carbohydrate-heavy first meals, protein does not interrupt metabolic balance or prematurely shift the body into storage mode.

Using Fasting to Support Healthy Eating

Fasting is not an extreme intervention, but a supportive eating plan that reinforces your healthy eating patterns. Periods of intentional food abstention reduce the constant digestive demands on your body and help restore sensitivity to natural hunger and fullness cues. Within this *Road Map,* fasting is understood primarily as a behavioral and neurological reset, particularly if you have a carbohydrate dependency. By creating space between impulse and action, fasting allows you to understand better your body's actual hunger signals rather than habitual eating patterns. It also helps your body cleanse itself at the cellular level. Fasting is most effective when eating periods that follow the fast emphasize protein-focused foods paired with healthy fats.

Two fasting approaches are presented as supportive tools within a healthy eating lifestyle: Intermittent Fasting and Alternate-Day Fasting. As with all aspects of this *Road Map*, individual circumstances vary, and guidance from one's primary care physician should be considered when determining how fasting may be applied along the journey.

Intermittent Fasting

Intermittent fasting, commonly practiced alongside daily eating windows, allows insulin levels to remain low for extended periods. This supports the body's ability to access stored energy rather than relying exclusively on incoming calories. Within this framework, eating patterns such as one meal a day (OMAD) or two meals a day (TMAD) provide practical structure. OMAD concentrates your daily nourishment into a single, intentional meal, while TMAD allows you two clearly defined meals within a limited window of time. Both approaches reduce constant digestive demands on your system and encourage purposeful eating rather than reactive eating.

For example, eating windows can significantly reduce snacking and grazing. By limiting your eating to defined periods, your body is no longer trained to expect food continuously. This reinforces the value of intentional meal timing and helps you distinguish between your body's actual hunger signals and those created by previous eating habits or environmental cues, e.g., seeing food advertisements.

For most people, intermittent fasting is best introduced gradually. A natural starting point is the overnight fast that occurs while you sleep. You can extend this fast by stopping your eating at least three hours before bedtime—which often improves sleep—and by waiting at least 90 minutes after waking before your first meal. For example, stopping at 9:00 p.m. and eating again at 9:00 a.m. creates a 12-hour fasting window. Even this simple starting point often leads to noticeable improvements in your appetite awareness.

Intermittent fasting can be understood as a form of metabolic healing when it is introduced gradually and practiced consistently. By extending the natural overnight fast, such as stopping eating earlier in the evening and delaying the first meal in the morning, you reduce constant insulin stimulation and give your body regular periods to rebalance how it processes and uses energy. Even modest fasting windows can begin restoring metabolic flexibility and improving how your body responds to food.

As your comfort with intermittent fasting increases, you can gradually increase the fasting window. This may involve delaying the first meal to be slightly later in the day and reducing the length of the eating window. These adjustments should be made progressively rather than abruptly, allowing your body and behavior patterns to adapt without undue stress.

Intermittent fasting can be practiced most days of the week rather than only occasionally. You technically fast each day while you sleep, but intermittent fasting is better understood as intentionally extending that fasting window before and/or after sleep. When you practice intermittent fasting consistently, you establish a metabolic rhythm and an easy-to-remember eating pattern, while occasional variations in timing help prevent your body from predicting your eating window and diminishing the benefits. When combined with nutrient-dense, protein-focused meals during eating periods, intermittent fasting supports healthy eating as a sustainable lifestyle rather than a short-term intervention.

Alternate Day Fasting

Alternate day fasting builds on the foundation you establish through intermittent fasting by introducing longer, less frequent fasting periods. Instead of focusing only on daily eating windows, you alternate days of intentional, structured eating with a complete 24-hour fast. When used selectively, this approach helps interrupt eating patterns your body may begin to anticipate through consistent routines, preserving the effectiveness of your fasting practices over time.

Alternate day fasting is not intended to compensate for overeating on your eating days. The goal of alternate day fasting is to extend the period during which your insulin levels remain low, allowing your body to rely more fully on stored energy. For some individuals, this may involve a complete fast supported by water and other non-caloric beverages. Plain water, mineral water, or unsweetened black coffee, black tea, or green tea can be consumed without breaking your fast and prevent feelings of total deprivation.

Alternate day fasting works like a brief move into the fast lane rather than a permanent lane change. It is not required for every journey, nor is it intended to replace your daily eating habits. When used thoughtfully and sparingly, it serves as a strategic tool that supports healthy eating by reinforcing discipline and giving your metabolism additional time to rest, reset, and support your body's natural repair processes.

Staying Hydrated

Fasting can lead to dehydration, so you need to drink plenty of fluids, especially water, during your fast. Maintaining your electrolyte balance can be accomplished in tandem with your fluid intake by adding salt or electrolyte formulations to your water, provided they contain no sugars or caloric sweeteners. Some commercially available zero-sugar electrolyte beverages, like Gatorade Zero (not regular Gatorade), can be part of your routine on fasting days. There are also commercially available liquid or powder electrolytes you add to water. Be sure, though, to avoid those that contain flavored additives and artificial sweeteners, as they may stimulate appetite and undermine the impact of your fast, even in the absence of calories.

Another popular hydration option is to make a hot or cold drink with lemon juice, water, and a zero-sugar sweetener like Stevia. Lemon water supports digestive processes, as its mild acidity can stimulate saliva and gastric secretions, helping prepare the digestive system for meals. For some individuals, this can improve digestive comfort when consumed before meals. Lemon water also provides you with vitamin C and plant compounds that support immune function and general cellular health.

Please Note: You can become dehydrated even on eating days if you eat less and, as a result, drink fewer fluids because you do not feel as thirsty. It is essential that you intentionally drink at least 64 ounces of water per day to help your body remain adequately hydrated and functioning well. Adequate hydration supports digestion, circulation, and metabolic processes, and it often improves how you feel overall while also supporting steady progress on your healthy eating journey.

Structuring Meals

Once your eating times and fasting patterns are established, the next step is learning how to structure your meals within those boundaries. Structuring meals is not about rigid rules or perfect portions. It is about approaching each meal intentionally so that how you eat supports your progress rather than undermines it.

A structured meal is a planned eating event, not something that happens accidentally or continuously. When you sit down to eat, you are choosing to eat on purpose rather than grazing throughout the day. In some dietary approaches, grazing was once encouraged to prevent hunger, but it keeps digestion and insulin activity elevated, making it difficult for you to recognize true hunger and fullness. Structured meals, by contrast, give your body clear signals about when nourishment begins and when it ends.

Whether you are eating one meal a day (OMAD) or two meals a day (TMAD), structure becomes even more critical as meal frequency decreases. Fewer meals do not mean casual meals. Each meal carries a greater responsibility to provide nourishment. Sitting down, slowing down, and ending the meal helps reinforce discipline and reduces the tendency to drift back into old habits.

How you eat during a meal matters just as much as what you eat. A straightforward practice to adopt is to take a bite of food, put down your fork or spoon, and thoroughly enjoy the taste before taking the next bite. This intentional pause gives your body time to signal fullness and increases satisfaction by allowing you to truly taste your food. Eating this way helps break the habit of rushing through meals, and it makes it easier for you to stop eating when you are satisfied rather than when your plate is empty.

Another practical strategy that supports attentiveness and awareness of feeling full is to place all available food on a serving platter and transfer only the amount you want to eat at that moment onto your plate. You then add more to your plate if genuine hunger remains. This approach counters the ingrained habit we were taught as kids to eat everything placed on our plates. But doing so often overrides your body's natural "I am full" signals. By starting with smaller portions and reassessing your hunger as you eat, you relearn how to recognize and respect when you feel full.

How you portion food also plays a role in structuring meals. Rather than loading your plate with everything you might eat, it is often more effective to begin with a reasonable portion, knowing you can add more if genuine hunger remains. This approach naturally slows the pace of eating and supports awareness. Eating until you are satisfied—not stuffed—helps you refrain from overeating just because food remains on your plate.

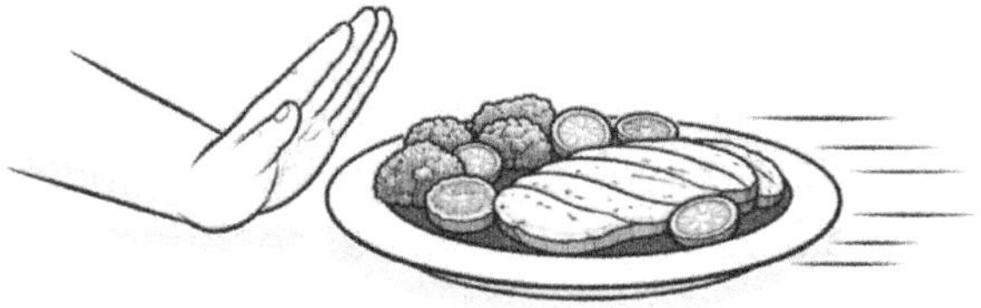

Finally, structuring meals includes learning how to end a meal deliberately. When you finish eating, clear the plate—saving what remains as leftovers if possible—step away from food, and mentally close the eating window. This simple action reinforces boundaries and reduces the temptation to keep eating out of habit rather than out of hunger.

Structuring meals is like learning how to drive smoothly once you are on the road. Timing tells you when to drive, but structure determines how safely and efficiently you travel. When your mealtimes are intentional, paced, and complete, healthy eating becomes easier to sustain and far less dependent on willpower alone.

Prioritizing Protein with Healthy Fats

Once meals are structured, the following rule of the road is deciding what forms the foundation of each meal. In this healthy eating *Road Map*, quality protein paired with healthy fats serves as the primary building block. This combination supports your feeling of fullness, stabilizes blood sugar, and provides the nutrients your body needs without creating unnecessary insulin spikes.

Protein is prioritized because it plays a central role in maintaining metabolic health. It supports muscle preservation, tissue repair, and overall strength. Muscle loss is a common concern with many eating plans, and protein is essential for building and maintaining muscle. When your meals are built around adequate protein, you are more likely to lose body fat while preserving muscle and less likely to experience persistent hunger, cravings, or the urge to snack between meals.

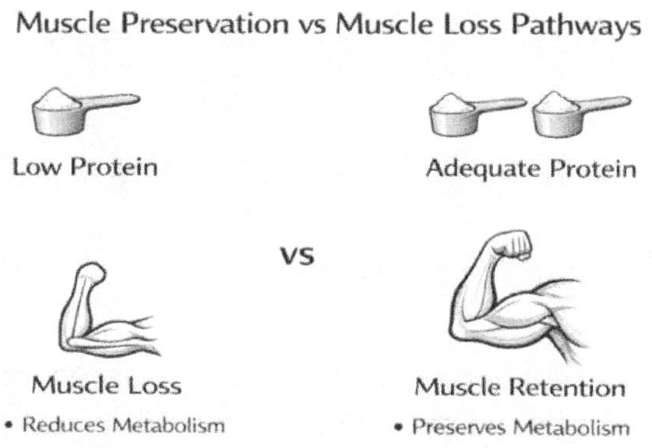

Healthy natural fats are intentionally paired with quality protein rather than treated as a stand-alone fuel source. When eaten together, fats slow digestion, help you feel full, and support appetite control. This pairing provides steadier energy and helps prevent the rapid rise and fall in blood sugar that often occurs with carbohydrate-heavy meals. Your goal is not to eat fat for its own sake, but to rely on the healthy fats that naturally accompany quality protein sources.

Prioritizing quality protein with healthy natural fats supports metabolic health by keeping insulin stimulation lower while still making meals satisfying. When insulin demand is lower, your body is better able to access stored energy between meals, making fasting periods easier to maintain and reducing the likelihood of overeating later in the day.

It should be noted that you do not need to add more fat to a high-quality protein that already contains fat. Healthy fats can be added, though, when the quality protein source is lean. Cooking lean protein with healthy fat should be sufficient to maintain the priorities of protein first, healthy fat to support the protein, and low-carbohydrate intake. You can think of it like an inverted pyramid in terms of priorities.

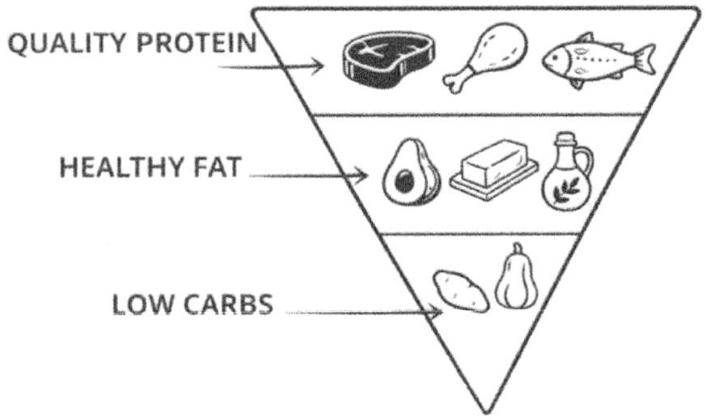

From a behavioral perspective, protein-centered meals also help reduce carbohydrate dependence. When meals consistently meet your body's nutritional needs, hunger becomes more stable, and eating is less driven by reward or emotion—food shifts from a constant source of stimulation to its proper role as nourishment.

Protein-rich, healthy fats occur naturally in minimally processed whole foods. These include fats found in animal-based proteins, natural oils derived from fruits such as olives and avocados, and traditional cooking fats that remain stable when heated, such as bacon grease. Specific food examples and practical guidance for choosing protein-containing healthy fats are addressed in greater detail in the chapter on "Foods to Eat."

These principles apply whether your eating plan is keto-style, carnivore-style, or a ketovore hybrid of the two. In each case, protein serves as the primary indicator of whether a meal is nutritionally sufficient. At the same time, fats are intentionally used to support that protein rather than dominate the meal's nutritional profile.

As your appetite becomes more regulated, you may feel satisfied with less food overall. While this is a positive outcome, it makes it especially important to ensure you are still eating enough protein. When eating windows narrow or fasting becomes more routine, under-eating protein is one of the most common mistakes. Prioritizing protein first at each meal helps protect lean muscle and supports fat loss rather than muscle loss.

Protein functions like the engine of your vehicle, while healthy fats provide steady fuel for the journey. When meals are built on this principle, eating becomes more straightforward, more satisfying, and easier to sustain. Over time, this approach supports healthy eating as a lasting lifestyle rather than a temporary strategy.

The 10:1 Protein Rule

You will notice in this book that I only discuss measuring fat, protein, and carbohydrates. In fact, calories are rarely mentioned at all, even though they are the focus of many eating plans. There is, however, one guideline you might consider when selecting or avoiding protein sources. This guideline is called the 10:1 Protein Rule.

This rule suggests that to determine if the food source is a healthy choice on your healthy eating journey, look at the ratio of calories to grams of protein in the food portion. The math can be easily done in your head without a calculator. Look at the nutritional label of the food, find the number of grams of protein in a serving, and add a zero to the end of that number. Now look at the number of calories on the nutritional label and see whether it is higher or lower than that number. If lower, it should be a good food choice. If it is significantly higher, you might not want to choose it. If close to the number, you can still consider eating it.

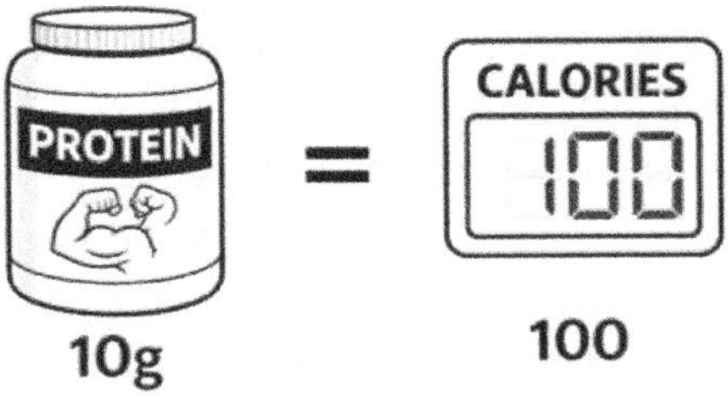

10:1 Protein-To-Calories Rule

One thing to note is that some nutritional labels can be deceiving. That is, the values listed are for a serving size, but what is the serving size? If it is a small amount and you tend to eat more than that, you would definitely want to avoid foods with more calories than protein. If the number is lower than the ratio value or close to it, you should be careful about how much you eat.

Managing Carbohydrates

Carbohydrates differ from protein and fat in how they affect your body. When you eat carbohydrates, blood glucose rises, and insulin is released. While insulin plays a necessary role in normal metabolism, frequent or excessive insulin stimulation makes it harder for your body to access stored energy. It can slow progress toward improved metabolic health. For this reason, carbohydrates are addressed after protein and fats, which provide nourishment without triggering the same insulin response.

Managing Carbohydrates Within Meals and Food Selections

A helpful approach to managing carbohydrates is to focus on total carbohydrates rather than net carbohydrates. Net carbohydrate calculations subtract fiber and sugar alcohols, which often creates confusion, and can help you observe how a food truly impacts your appetite and insulin signaling. Looking at total carbohydrates provides a more straightforward, more consistent way to evaluate foods without performing calculations or searching for net carbohydrate values on labels.

Managing carbohydrates then shifts from evaluating individual foods to understanding proportions at the meal level. When carbohydrates crowd out protein, hunger often returns quickly, cravings increase, and energy becomes less stable. When you eat protein first and allow carbohydrates, if included, to remain secondary, meals are more satisfying, and appetite becomes easier to regulate. This sequence helps you feel full after eating and reduces the likelihood of overeating later in the day.

How you manage carbohydrates will vary based on your chosen eating approach. In a keto-style framework, carbohydrates are kept very low to minimize insulin stimulation. In a carnivore-style framework, carbohydrates may be nearly absent. In hybrid whole-food approaches, carbohydrates may still appear, but in limited amounts and carefully selected. In each case, the guiding principle remains the same: carbohydrates are optional and supportive, not primary.

Clear boundaries around carbohydrate intake help remove guesswork and reduce decision fatigue. Instead of negotiating carbohydrate choices at every meal, defined guidelines allow you to eat with confidence and consistency. This structure supports long-term adherence to healthy eating far more effectively than relying solely on willpower.

A suggested amount of carbohydrates to allow yourself to eat per day is between 20 and 30, but no more than 40 to 50.

As your appetite stabilizes and metabolic health improves, your desire for carbohydrates often diminishes naturally. This change is not forced, but rather a response to meals that are more satisfying and nourishing. By managing carbohydrates thoughtfully, you align your food choices with how your body functions best and support steady, sustainable progress.

Within the *Road Map,* carbohydrates function like side roads rather than main highways. You may use them selectively and intentionally, but they no longer determine the direction of your journey. When managed well, carbohydrates stop controlling your eating decisions and allow healthy eating to remain calm, focused, and sustainable over time.

Considering Supplements Carefully

Supplements occupy a supportive role within a healthy eating lifestyle. They are not a substitute for healthy eating, structured meals, fasting practices, or prioritizing protein with healthy fats. Instead, supplements are best viewed as optional tools that may provide incremental benefit once the foundational principles of this journey are already in place.

For my own healthy eating journey, I found only certain supplements consistently helpful to me daily (your experience may be different). The first is raw apple cider vinegar with the mother; the second is an olive oil supplement; and the third contains omega fatty acids 3, 6, 7, and 9, including turmeric. I found these three supplements enhanced the development of healthy eating patterns.

These three supplements can be consumed in various forms. The amount to take from each one is as follows:

- One tablespoon of raw apple cider vinegar with the mother, or one powdered capsule, taken in the morning and the evening. I found the Herbtonics Raw Apple Cider Vinegar Capsules 1500mg with Mother to be a good choice, and it is available on Amazon: https://edcot.info/apple-cider-vinegar.
- One tablespoon of extra virgin cold-pressed olive oil, or one softgel capsule, taken in the morning and the evening. I found the Healthy Origins Extra Virgin Olive Oil 1,250 mg to be a good choice, and it is available on Amazon: https://edcot.info/olive-oil.
- One omega-3 fatty acid capsule that includes turmeric, taken in the morning and the evening. I found the Livingood Daily Omega 3 6 9 Plus Turmeric Curcumin – Omega 3 Supplement to be a good choice, and it is available on Amazon: https://edcot.info/omega3-turmeric.

I found the softgel and capsule forms easier to consume consistently and at the appropriate times of day. This is especially the case when taken during fasting periods, as they allow supplementation without disrupting eating windows or undermining the metabolic benefits carried over from the previous day before eating again.

Many health advisors recommend additional supplements for a wide range of purposes, from metabolic support to inflammation management to general wellness. While some of these may be appropriate in specific circumstances, the number of available options can quickly become overwhelming. Taken together, supplements can also become expensive, with monthly costs adding up rapidly. It is entirely possible to “pickle yourself” in supplements—and strain your budget—without experiencing benefits proportional to the effort or expense. I found taking too many supplements had little impact on my healthy eating progress, but definitely impacted my wallet!

Restraint and discernment are therefore essential. Supplements should be added selectively, one at a time, and only when there is a clear purpose for their use. More is not better. In many cases, consistent improvements in eating timing, food quality, protein intake, and carbohydrate management produce far greater results than adding another supplement.

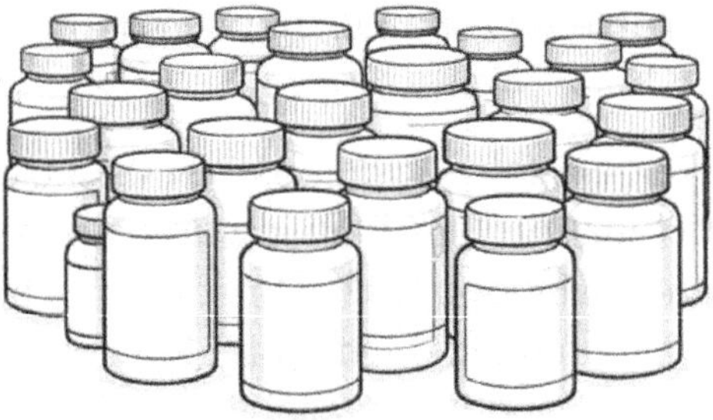

It is also essential that supplements be approached with appropriate medical oversight. Any supplement should be discussed with and approved by your primary care physician, particularly if you have existing health conditions or are taking prescribed medications. If any supplement causes discomfort, digestive upset, or other adverse effects, it should be discontinued. A supplement that interferes with how you feel or function is not supporting your journey, regardless of its perceived benefits.

Supplements are like optional accessories rather than essential vehicle components. They may enhance comfort or performance in certain situations, but the journey itself depends on how you drive, the route you follow, and how consistently you apply the rules of the road. When used carefully and conservatively, supplements can play a small, supportive role—but they should never become the focus of a healthy eating lifestyle.

Key Points to Remember from Chapter 3

The following key points from Chapter 3 serve as road signs to guide your progress on your healthy eating lifestyle journey.

- Healthy eating works best when you understand that progress happens both internally and externally, with improvements in metabolism and visceral fat reduction occurring alongside visible changes on the scale and in the mirror.
- When you eat matters, because defined eating times and intentional fasting help your body regulate insulin and support better metabolic health.
- Hydration is vital in a healthy eating lifestyle. Be sure to drink enough water and fluids with electrolytes throughout the day. Lemon water is a good digestive option to consider as well.
- Protein should anchor each meal, with healthy fats supporting it so you feel full, protect muscle, and support fat loss as eating windows narrow.
- Carbohydrates work best when they support protein rather than dominate the meal, generally staying within about ten grams of total carbohydrates for every one gram of protein, so they do not drive your food choices.
- Supplements can be helpful, and a few are, but be careful about how many others you take.

- Clear boundaries and steady habits matter more than perfection, making healthy eating easier to maintain through structure instead of willpower.

Chapter 4: Foods to Eat

Knowing the Approved Lanes

"He makes grass grow for the cattle, and plants for man to cultivate—bringing forth food from the earth." – Psalm 104:14-15a (NIV)

Chapter 4 shifts the focus from principles to practical choices by helping you identify foods that support steady progress on your journey. Within the *Road Map* metaphor, these foods function as approved lanes—options that let you move forward with fewer detours and unnecessary side trips. The emphasis here is not on trends or perfection, but on making consistent, informed choices that work with your body rather than against it.

Priority in your personal healthy eating plan is given to organically produced, grass-fed, free-range foods, and, when selecting fish, to fresh, wild-caught varieties. When these food options are limited, inaccessible, or unaffordable, commonly available alternatives are still acceptable choices. The goal is not exclusivity in food sourcing, but nourishment. Your focus is on selecting foods that are satisfying, minimally processed, free from unnecessary additives and preservatives, and—most importantly—foods you will genuinely enjoy eating.

While many dieting plans focus first on what to avoid eating, the *Road Map* focuses first on what you will want to choose to eat to support your healthy eating lifestyle. This includes identifying healthy meats and fish, fruits and vegetables, acceptable whole grains, rice, and nuts; the importance of eggs, whole milk, and other dairy products; healthy oils and fats; and which spices, condiments, and sweeteners are nutritious.

Please Note: You will notice some commonly accepted "diet foods" are intentionally absent from the Foods to Eat. Many products marketed as healthy or low-calorie either contain more sugar than expected or rely on heavy processing, artificial ingredients, and refined substitutes. While these foods may appear supportive on the surface, their composition can interfere with how your body produces and uses energy at the cellular level.

Certain ingredients found in traditional diet foods can disrupt normal cellular function, including the mitochondria—the structures within your cells that produce energy. When this cellular process is impaired, progress may stall despite good intentions, calorie control, or adherence to "diet-approved" labels. By excluding these foods, this *Road Map* reinforces that lasting progress is built on nourishment that supports cellular health, not on products designed to imitate healthy eating without truly sustaining it.

Together, the choices presented here provide a clear and usable framework for food selection, equipping you to make daily decisions that sustain momentum and reinforce long-term healthy eating habits.

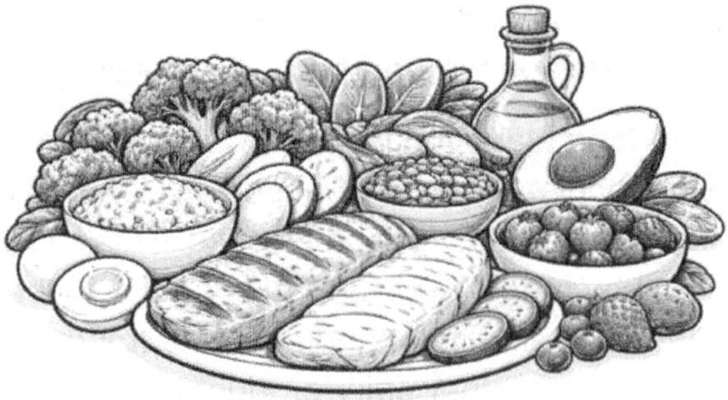

Meats, Fish, and Poultry

The following list identifies healthy types of meat and fish that are rich in protein, support a feeling of fullness, help preserve muscle, and promote metabolic stability when minimally processed and responsibly sourced. Many of these foods naturally contain healthy fats that contribute to satiety and sustained energy.

Recommended Meats

For canned meats, choose options with simple ingredients such as meat and salt, and avoid products that include fillers, sweeteners, seed oils, or modified starches.

- Bacon Ends (uncured, sugar-free, verify ingredients)
- Bacon Pieces (uncured, sugar-free, verify ingredients)
- Bacon, Beef (uncured, sugar-free, pasture-raised, or grass-fed)
- Bacon, Pork (uncured, sugar-free, pasture-raised)
- Beef Brisket (grass-fed)
- Beef Brisket (grass-fed)
- Beef Chuck Roast (grass-fed)
- Beef Flank Steak (grass-fed)
- Beef Ground Hamburger (not overly lean, grass-fed)
- Beef Liver (grass-fed; used occasionally)
- Beef Ribeye Steak (grass-fed)
- Beef Shank (grass-fed)

- Beef Short Ribs (grass-fed)
- Beef Sirloin (grass-fed)
- Beef Skirt Steak (grass-fed)
- Bison (pasture-raised)
- Bison (pasture-raised)
- Chuck Roast (grass-fed)
- Elk (wild or pasture-raised)
- Goat (grass-fed or pasture-raised)
- Ground Hamburger (not lean, grass-fed)
- Lamb (grass-fed)
- Lamb (grass-fed)
- Pork Belly (pasture-raised)
- Pork Chops (pasture-raised)
- Pork Chops (pasture-raised)
- Pork Ribs (pasture-raised)
- Pork Shoulder (pasture-raised)
- Pork Shoulder (pasture-raised)
- Pork Tenderloin (pasture-raised)
- Ribeye Steak (grass-fed)
- Venison (wild or pasture-raised)

Recommended Fish

Salmon is a particularly valuable choice because it is rich in omega-3 fatty acids, which support heart health and reduce inflammation. When sourced as wild-caught, salmon also provides a natural balance of protein and healthy fats that help you feel full and sustain energy. For canned fish, select varieties packed in water or olive oil, and check labels to ensure no seed oils, sugars, or flavoring additives are included.

- Cod, Atlantic (wild caught)
- Cod, Pacific (wild caught)
- Halibut, Atlantic (wild caught)
- Halibut, Pacific (wild caught)
- Mackerel (wild caught)
- Salmon, Coho (wild caught)
- Salmon, King/Chinook (wild caught)
- Salmon, Pink (wild caught)
- Salmon, Sockeye (wild caught)
- Sardines (wild caught)
- Tuna, Albacore (wild caught; use in moderation)
- Tuna, Skipjack (wild caught; preferred for regular use)
- Tuna, Yellowfin (wild caught; use in moderation)

Recommended Shellfish

Shellfish can be included as acceptable options when prepared without sauces. However, they are generally best consumed occasionally rather than relied upon as primary protein sources, especially for those seeking tighter appetite or carbohydrate control. For shellfish, choose fresh or frozen options with no added ingredients whenever possible. If packaged or canned, review the ingredient list to ensure it contains only shellfish, water, or salt, and avoid products with added sugars, breading, sauces, or seed oils.

- Blue Crab (wild caught)
- Caribbean Lobster (wild caught, not farm-raised)
- Dungeness Crab (wild caught)
- European Lobster (wild caught, not farm-raised)
- King Crab (wild caught)
- Lobster, American (wild caught)
- Maine Lobster / American Lobster (wild caught, not farm-raised)
- Oysters (wild caught)
- Rock Lobster / Spiny Lobster (wild caught, not farm-raised)
- Scallops, Sea (wild caught)
- Shrimp, Gulf or Cold-Water (wild caught)
- Snow Crab (wild caught)

Recommended Poultry

Dark poultry meats are preferable to white breast meat alone, as they naturally contain more fat, which helps you feel full and sustain energy.

- Chicken Breast (free range)
- Chicken Thighs (free range)
- Chicken, Whole (free range)
- Cornish Hen (free range)
- Duck (free range or wild)

- Goose (free range)
- Guinea Fowl (free range or wild)
- Pheasant (free range or wild)
- Quail (free range or wild)
- Turkey Breast (free range)
- Turkey Drumsticks (free range)
- Turkey Legs (free range)
- Turkey Thighs (free range)
- Turkey, Ground (free range)

Fruits and Vegetables

This list focuses on fruits and vegetables that complement a healthy eating lifestyle by providing essential nutrients, fiber, and variety, while avoiding unnecessary spikes in blood sugar. The selections emphasize whole, minimally processed plant foods, as their liquid forms, such as juices, often concentrate sugars and do not provide the same feeling of fullness as eating the whole food. Because fruits and some vegetables contain natural amounts of carbohydrates, portion size and frequency matter, and these foods are most supportive when selected with that in mind rather than eaten in unlimited quantities.

Recommended Fruits

Moderation in the amounts of fruits eaten is an important consideration. Some berries, like blueberries, contain more natural sugar that can disrupt your progress. Other common fruits like apples, bananas, grapes, and melons, to name a few, contain high amounts of sugar that can also hinder your progress. Those fruits, therefore, fall into the Foods to Avoid category and will be covered in that chapter. For canned fruit, avoid products packed in syrup or juice concentrate and choose only those packed in water, recognizing that fresh fruit is generally preferable.

- Avocado
- Black Olives (brined)
- Blackberries
- Blueberries
- Castelvetrano Olives (brined)
- Green Olives (brined)
- Kalamata Olives (brined)
- Lemons
- Lemon Water (hot or cold)
- Limes
- Raspberries
- Strawberries
- Stuffed Olives (brined, stuffed with pimento)

Recommended Vegetables

Moderation is also important with certain vegetables that contain higher natural sugar content. Yellow and orange bell peppers, for example, are higher in sugar than green peppers and are best eaten in moderation. Similarly, cherry and grape tomatoes contain more concentrated sugars than larger tomato varieties and are easier to overconsume. For canned vegetables, review ingredient and nutrition labels to confirm they contain only the vegetable itself, water, or salt, and are free from added sugars, starches, or preservatives.

When cooking vegetables, using healthy fats such as olive oil, avocado oil, butter, or ghee can improve flavor, support satiety, and enhance the absorption of fat-soluble nutrients. Vegetables can also be cooked in the natural fat left in the pan after cooking beef, chicken, or bacon, providing a stable, traditional cooking fat while adding flavor.

- Asparagus
- Bok Choy (and related Asian cabbages)
- Broccoli
- Brussels Sprouts
- Butter Lettuce
- Button Mushrooms (White)
- Cauliflower
- Celery
- Cremini Mushrooms (Baby Bella)
- Cucumbers
- Garlic
- Green Beans
- Green Bell Pepper (preferred)
- Green Cabbage
- Kale
- Mixed Greens Lettuce
- Orange Bell Pepper (in moderation)
- Portobello Mushrooms
- Red Cabbage (Purple)
- Red Onions

- Romaine Lettuce
- Shiitake Mushrooms
- Spaghetti Squash (in moderation)
- Spinach (fresh or lightly cooked)
- Vidalia Onions (use sparingly due to higher natural sugar)
- White Onions
- Yellow Bell Pepper (in moderation)
- Yellow Onions
- Zucchini

Whole Grains, Rice, and Nuts

Rice and whole grains are omitted here, and their omission is intentional. These foods tend to have a greater impact on blood sugar and appetite regulation than the foods listed here and are addressed later in the *Road Map*.

Nuts are included with caution because they are calorie-dense, easy to overconsume, and more likely to stimulate appetite than promote lasting satiety. While they contain beneficial fats, their carbohydrate content and frequent exposure to seed oils during processing make them best used intentionally and in limited amounts rather than as everyday staples.

Recommended Nuts

The following nuts are generally lower in net carbohydrates and have more favorable fat profiles when consumed in small portions. These are best eaten occasionally, preferably with meals rather than as standalone snacks.

- Brazil Nuts (raw, dry roasted, lightly salted or unsalted)
- Cashews (in small quantities)
- Chestnuts (in small amounts)
- Macadamia Nuts (raw, dry roasted, lightly salted or unsalted)
- Pecans (raw, dry roasted, lightly salted or unsalted)
- Pistachios (in small quantities)
- Walnuts (raw, dry roasted, lightly salted or unsalted)

Eggs, Milk, and Other Dairy Products

Eggs, milk, and other dairy products can support a healthy eating lifestyle when they are minimally processed and well-tolerated by your body. They provide high-quality protein, natural fats, and key nutrients that promote satiety and metabolic stability. Because tolerance to dairy varies, these foods are best chosen intentionally, favoring full-fat options with simple ingredients, and using your body's response as the primary guide to eating them.

Recommended Eggs

Eggs, once widely discouraged due to concerns about cholesterol and heart health, are now recognized as a healthy food option based on more recent research. They are a highly nutritious whole-food choice that can play an essential role in a balanced eating plan. The color of the eggshell—brown or white—does not significantly impact the nutritional value of the egg. What matters most is how the hens are raised and what they are fed. But if you have a preference—select it! For packaged or liquid egg products, confirm that the ingredients list includes only eggs, without added oils, stabilizers, or flavoring agents. The following types of eggs are your preferred choices.

- Brown Eggs (any size; pasture-raised or free range)
- Brown Eggs, Organic (any size; pasture-raised or free range)
- White Eggs (any size; pasture-raised or free range)
- White Eggs, Organic (any size; pasture-raised or free range)

Recommended Milk

Milk and cream products can be supportive when they are well tolerated and chosen with attention to fat content and ingredient simplicity. Low-fat and fat-free milk products are generally not recommended for this healthy eating lifestyle, as removing fat reduces feelings of fullness and often coincides with higher lactose impact and added stabilizers. Full-fat options are more satisfying and align better with metabolic stability. For powdered milk, carefully review ingredients for added sugars, fillers, or highly processed components, as these products are more likely to include them.

For coffee and tea, whole milk, half-and-half, and heavy whipping cream may be used in small amounts when well tolerated. These options are generally more satisfying than low-fat alternatives and are less likely to trigger cravings. Sweetened creamers and flavored milk products are best avoided, as they often contain added sugars, seed oils, or thickeners that can undermine your metabolic stability. The recommended milk products are as follows.

- Coconut Milk (canned, free of seed oils and gums, used sparingly)
- Goat Milk (whole, plain; used sparingly)
- Half-and-Half (with simple ingredients)
- Heavy Whipping Cream (no added thickeners)
- Sheep's Milk (whole, plain; used sparingly)
- Whole Milk (organic and grass-fed when available)

Recommended Cheese

For cheese, choose full-fat varieties with minimal ingredients, ideally limited to milk, cultures, salt, and enzymes, and avoid products with added starches, gums, or seed oils. These cheeses are best selected in block or wheel form, with ingredient lists limited to milk, cultures, salt, and enzymes. Aged cheeses are often better tolerated because they have lower lactose content. Also note that cheeses from New Zealand have had to meet stricter ingredient quality requirements and are often the better choice (some are packaged in the USA but made in New Zealand).

- Blue Cheese
- Brie
- Camembert
- Cheddar (full-fat, aged)
- Goat Cheese (minimal ingredients)
- Gouda
- Gruyère
- Mozzarella (fresh, full-fat)
- Parmesan (aged)

- Provolone
- Sheep's Milk Cheeses (such as Manchego)
- Swiss

Recommended Cottage Cheese

Cottage cheese is best selected with higher milk-fat content, as low-fat versions are often less satisfying and may contain added ingredients to compensate for the reduced fat. Check cottage cheese for added sugars, fruit concentrates, thickeners, or flavorings—favor plain, full-fat options with short ingredient lists. Acceptable cottage cheese options are as follows.

- Cottage Cheese, Plain (4% milk fat or higher; whole milk, small or large curd)
- Cottage Cheese, Unsweetened (4% milk fat or higher; whole milk, small or large curd)

Recommended Yogurt

Low-fat and fat-free yogurts are generally not recommended for this healthy eating lifestyle, as removing fat often reduces feelings of fullness and is usually offset by added sugars, starches, or flavorings. Full-fat yogurt is more satisfying than low-fat varieties, supports steadier energy, and aligns better with the emphasis on whole, minimally processed foods. For yogurt, check for added sugars, fruit concentrates, thickeners, or flavorings, and favor plain, full-fat options with short ingredient lists. Acceptable yogurt options are as follows.

- Goat's Milk Yogurt (plain, full-fat)
- Greek Yogurt (plain, full-fat)
- Sheep's Milk Yogurt (plain, full-fat)

- Skyr (plain, full-fat)
- Yogurt, Plain (full-fat, made from whole milk)

Healthy Oils

Healthy oils support metabolic stability and overall health when used appropriately. In recent years, greater attention has been given to the type and processing of fats used in everyday cooking, leading to a growing recognition that not all oils function the same way in the body. While earlier dietary guidance often emphasized replacing animal fats with industrial seed oils, emerging understanding has highlighted the importance of choosing stable, minimally processed oils instead of the more common seed oils. The concerns surrounding seed oils and why they are best avoided are addressed more fully in the "Foods to Avoid" chapter.

Oil selection plays a vital role in supporting a healthy eating lifestyle. Naturally derived, minimally processed oils that are less prone to oxidation are better choices for cooking and food preparation, as they remain more stable when heated and during long-term storage. Healthy fats found in oils such as cold-pressed extra virgin olive oil, avocado oil, coconut oil, and MCT oil provide a reliable source of fuel and support satiety and metabolic stability. Packaging also matters; oils stored in dark glass containers are better protected from exposure to light, which helps slow oxidation and reduces the risk of the oil becoming rancid before it is used.

Recommended Oils

The following oils are more stable, less processed, and better aligned with metabolic health than industrial seed oils.

- Avocado Oil (cold-pressed or expeller-pressed; suitable for higher-heat cooking)

- Coconut Oil (virgin or unrefined; stable for cooking and baking)
- Extra Virgin Olive Oil (cold-pressed, unrefined; best for low-heat cooking and dressings)
- MCT Oil (derived from coconut oil; typically used uncooked or added after cooking)

Recommended Fats

The following fats are also commonly used in cooking and align with the same stability principles as the healthy oils listed above.

- Beef Fat or Tallow (from grass-fed or pasture-raised sources; stable for higher-heat cooking)
- Butter (grass-fed or pasture-raised cows when available; suitable for low to moderate heat)
- Ghee (clarified butter; grass-fed or pasture-raised sources when available, higher smoke point)
- Chick Fat (schmaltz/rendered chicken fat from drippings; free-range or pasture-raised)
- Duck Fat (from drippings; free-range or pasture-raised)

It should be noted that olives, which appear under Fruits above, are valued primarily for their fat content, but using them in moderation is essential, as they contain various amounts of sugar.

Spices, Condiments, and Sweeteners

Most spices can be used freely without negatively affecting metabolic health, while many condiments contain hidden ingredients that can hinder progress.

Natural sweeteners are also addressed. After years of consuming refined sugars, it is natural to experience cravings for sweetness as your eating preferences shift. Natural sweeteners can help bridge this transition by satisfying cravings while supporting metabolic health. These alternatives are typically used more sparingly, place less immediate demand on insulin regulation, and help promote steadier energy levels and improved feelings of fullness throughout the day. Used wisely, natural sweeteners can support consistency without derailing progress.

Recommended Spices

Most spices may be used liberally, individually, or in combination, provided they are pure and free from added sugars, starches, or fillers. When possible, choose single-ingredient spices rather than blends. If you do choose a blend, be sure it contains no sugar or anti-caking agents. The following list of spices is not intended to be comprehensive, but rather to highlight those commonly used, widely available, and easy to incorporate into everyday cooking. *Many additional spices may also be used, provided they are whole or minimally processed, and align with the same principles outlined in this chapter.*

- Basil (dried or fresh)
- Black Pepper (freshly ground, coarse or fine)
- White Pepper (milder flavor than black pepper)
- Cayenne Pepper (use sparingly)
- Chili Powder (mild or hot)
- Cinnamon (Ceylon preferred when available)
- Coriander (ground or whole seed)
- Cumin (ground or whole seed)

- Garlic (fresh cloves)
- Garlic Powder (fine or granulated)
- Garlic Salt (combined seasoning; use to taste)
- Ginger (fresh or ground)
- Nutmeg (use sparingly)
- Onion (fresh)
- Onion Powder (fine or granulated)
- Onion Salt (combined seasoning; use to taste)
- Oregano (dried or fresh)
- Paprika (sweet or smoked)
- Rosemary (dried or fresh)
- Sage (dried or fresh)
- Sea Salt (use to taste)
- Himalayan Salt (used to taste)
- Thyme (dried or fresh)

Recommended Condiments

Condiments can either support a healthy eating lifestyle or quietly work against it, depending on what they contain. Many store-bought options include added sugars, seed oils, or preservatives that disrupt your metabolic balance and trigger food cravings. For that reason, condiments are best used as minimal accents chosen carefully. When possible, homemade versions—especially mayonnaise, dressings, and sauces—are encouraged, as they avoid problematic ingredients and let you add flavor without undermining your health goals. The following condiments are generally supportive when the ingredient list is simple and the portions are reasonable.

- Aioli (olive oil–based, homemade or clean commercial versions)
- Coconut Aminos (used sparingly)
- Hot Sauce (simple ingredients, heat from peppers without sugar)
- Mayonnaise (made with olive oil or avocado oil)
- Yellow Mustard (classic yellow mustard when plain, without added sugar)
- Dijon Mustard (traditional Dijon-style without added sugar)
- Ground Mustard (stone ground, whole grain, or whole seed with simple acceptable ingredients)
- Brown Mustard (spicy or deli-style with no added sugar)
- Pesto (made with olive oil, herbs, and nuts)
- Pickles (made without added sugar and only simple ingredients)
- Salsa (fresh or refrigerated varieties with minimal ingredients)
- Apple Cider Vinegar, Raw with the Mother
- Balsamic Vinegar (used sparingly)
- Red Wine Vinegar (naturally fermented)
- White Wine Vinegar (naturally fermented)

Recommended Sweeteners

After years of regular sugar intake, it is normal for you to still crave sweet foods as your eating habits change. When chosen carefully and used sparingly, certain natural, nonsugar sweeteners can help ease the transition to healthier options with less impact on your blood sugar. Even powdered versions can be acceptable, but ingredient labels should always be checked to ensure they remain aligned with the principles of a healthy eating lifestyle.

Honey, even when raw or unprocessed, is still a concentrated source of sugar and can affect blood sugar and appetite regulation. While tiny amounts may be used rarely, most people experience greater metabolic benefit by avoiding honey altogether.

Sweeteners are most often added to coffee or tea, typically alongside milk or cream. When sweetness is desired, a small amount of stevia, monk fruit, or allulose can be used to gradually reduce the need for it, rather than maintaining a daily habit of sweetened beverages.

The following sweeteners may be used in small amounts to support the transition away from refined sugars.

- Allulose (granulated or powdered, use sparingly and with personal tolerance)
- Honey (raw, unprocessed varieties, use only occasionally and in tiny amounts)
- Molasses (blackstrap only, containing trace minerals like iron and magnesium, use only occasionally and in tiny amounts)
- Monk Fruit (liquid extract or powdered form)
- Stevia (liquid extract or powdered form)
- Stevia–Monk Fruit Blends (liquid or powdered simple blends)

Key Points to Remember from Chapter 4

The following key points from Chapter 4 serve as road signs to guide your progress on your healthy eating lifestyle journey.

- Choose foods that consistently support metabolic stability and feelings of fullness rather than foods driven by trends, marketing claims, or convenience alone.
- Prioritize whole, minimally processed foods, recognizing that sourcing and preparation matter.
- Build meals around protein-rich foods, using fruits and vegetables intentionally with awareness of their carbohydrate content, portion size, and your metabolic response.
- Include milk, cheeses, and other dairy products selectively, guided by your body's tolerance for them.
- Select healthy fats and stable oils like Avocado, Coconut, and Olive Oil as dependable fuel sources, taking care to monitor their quality and packaging to avoid becoming rancid.
- Use spices to enhance flavor, choose condiments carefully, and rely on simple ingredient lists rather than packaged convenience products.
- Treat natural sweeteners as transitional tools, using them sparingly and intentionally with the long-term goal of reducing your reliance on them.
- Focus on satisfying, easy-to-prepare meals to encourage long-term progress in developing your healthy eating lifestyle.

Chapter 5: Foods to Avoid

Avoiding the Closed Roads

"Everything is permissible for me,' but not everything is beneficial. 'Everything is permissible for me,' but I will not be mastered by anything" – 1 Corinthians 6:12 (NIV)

Every eating plan has foods to avoid that impede your progress toward your healthy eating goals. The *Road Map to a Healthy Eating Lifestyle* is no different. Just as construction zones and closed sections of a highway can delay or completely derail your travel plans, certain foods can disrupt your progress toward metabolic health. Some of the foods identified in Chapter 5 may be unexpected, as they are often considered acceptable—or even encouraged—in other eating plans. However, restoring and maintaining a healthy eating lifestyle requires recognizing that these foods interfere with progress at the metabolic level—how your body responds to them—not simply because of what they contain. These foods can be thought of as detours and closed roads, seen as obstacles that can prevent you from making progress toward your healthy eating destination.

One key reason to avoid certain foods is the amount of naturally occurring sugar they contain. Sugars are quickly absorbed and often trigger rapid spikes and drops in blood glucose. These spikes and drops can lead to fatigue and food cravings. Other foods common to other eating plans are included on this list because of what happens to your body at the cellular level. At this deeper level, some foods do disrupt the conditions the body relies upon for cellular maintenance, cleanup, and repair. These foods can promote inflammation, oxidative stress, and unstable glucose and insulin levels, hindering the body's ability to restore itself efficiently. Over time, that disruption can reduce or slow the body's normal renewal processes, making progress more complex to achieve and more challenging to maintain. Recognizing this cellular impact helps explain why some of the formerly acceptable foods are on the list of foods to avoid when following the *Road Map*.

When I began my own journey using the *Road Map*, I ate some of these foods consistently, especially Russet and baked sweet potatoes (sometimes also called yams in the USA). While I made progress on my healthy eating journey, it was not until I stopped eating these foods that my progress increased significantly. Though some of the health advisors I encountered on my journey had differing opinions on these foods, I ultimately found that some could be eaten *only rarely or in moderation.* At the start of your journey, including these foods in your eating plan, even in moderation, can encourage you to get started. Later, once you are more established on your journey, you can eliminate them. Keep in mind that eliminating them during your journey does not mean you can never eat them ever again! Instead, you will discover that they can be the occasional treat rather than a daily staple in your eating plan.

A prime example is when seasonal fruits and vegetables become available. Some of the hardest seasonal fruits and vegetables for me to avoid are apples, cherries, fresh corn, melons (both watermelon and cantaloupe), and grapes. Rather than feel deprived when they become available, I choose to eat them in moderation and try to select organically grown produce to minimize or eliminate exposure to contaminants and pesticides. When you naturally begin eating smaller portions, you purchase less food overall, making organic produce far more affordable and often reducing strain on your grocery budget compared to your prior spending patterns.

Again, if you choose to eat any of the foods on this list, do so rarely and in moderation. Your primary goal should be to maintain a healthy eating lifestyle. Allowing yourself to eat these foods—reintroducing them more often once you reach your destination—can eliminate feelings of deprivation and the urge to abandon healthy eating altogether. You do not want to be headed in the wrong direction with your food choices. Instead, think in terms of: "Let them eat cake (as long as it's keto)."

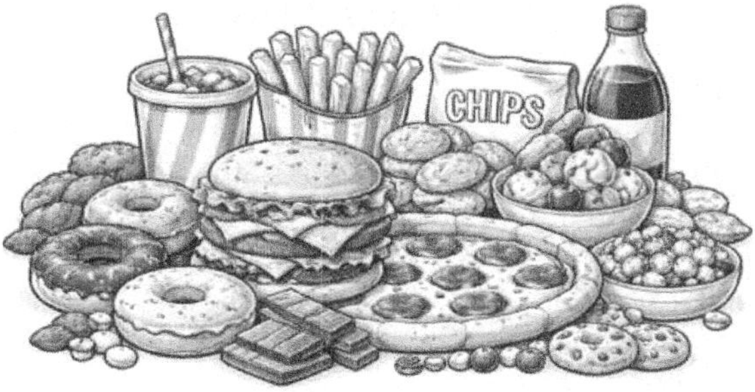

Meats, Fish, and Poultry to Avoid

Some meats, fish, and poultry are included here not because they are animal-based, but because their processing methods, additives, sourcing, and preparation transform them into foods that undermine your metabolic health. If you select to eat or them, do so in moderation and infrequently.

Meats to Avoid

- Bacon, Cured with Honey or Sugar
- Deli Meats (a processed meat)
- Ham Cured with Honey or Sugar
- Hot Dogs

- Lunch Meats (a processed meat)
- Meat, Battered
- Meat, Breaded
- Meat, Cured with Honey or Maple Sugar
- Meat, Low-Fat or Diet Varieties (often engineered as ultra-lean)
- Processed Meats (all types)
- Sausages (a processed meat)

Fish to Avoid

- Breaded Fish
- Cured Fish (containing added sugars)
- Farm-Raised Fish (especially salmon, tilapia, catfish)
- Fish Sticks
- Fried Fish
- Imitation Carb
- Processed Seafoods (all product types)
- Seafood Patties
- Smoked Fish (containing added sugars)

Shellfish to Avoid

Shellfish to avoid are those that contain fillers, starches, sugars, preservatives, and/or are battered in flour and fried in seed oils. The types of shellfish in this list include shrimp, oysters, clams, scallops, and calamari.

- Battered Shellfish (coated in flour and fried in seed oils)
- Breaded Shellfish (coated in flour or made with seed oils)
- Fried Shellfish (coated in flour or fried in seed oils)
- Heavily Seasoned Shellfish (containing sugars, seed oil, or preservatives)
- Imitation Crab
- Imitation Lobster
- Imitation Shellfish Products (made from processed fish, starches, sugars, and/or additives)
- Mixed Seafood Blends (containing starches, fillers, sugars, and/or seed oils)
- Pre-Marinated Shellfish (containing sugars, preservatives and/or seed oil)
- Processed Shellfish Products (all types)
- Seafood Cakes
- Seafood Patties
- Shellfish Packed in Industrial Oils or Sauces (canned or packaged in seed oils and/or sweetened sauces)
- Shellfish with Honey, Syrups, Sweet Sauces

Poultry to Avoid

Poultry should be avoided that contains fillers, starches, sugars, preservatives, and/or is battered in flour and fried in seed oils.

- Battered Chicken

- Battered Turkey
- Breaded Poultry (all varieties)
- Chicken Deli Meats
- Chicken Nuggets
- Chicken Patties
- Chicken Sausages
- Chicken Tenders
- Fried Chicken
- Fried Poultry (all varieties)
- Fried Turkey
- Pre-Marinated Poultry (made with seed oils, sugars, or flavor enhancers)
- Processed Poultry Products
- Sweetened or Glazed Poultry (prepared with honey, sugar, syrups, or sweet sauces)
- Ultra Lean or "Diet" Poultry Products (relying on additives)

Fruits and Vegetables to Avoid

Most of the listed fruits are high in natural sugars that can overwhelm metabolic regulation when consumed regularly. Even whole fruits deliver concentrated fructose and glucose that stimulate insulin secretion, increase appetite, and interfere with metabolic repair, especially for individuals working to restore insulin sensitivity. While fruit is often perceived as harmless or universally healthy, frequent intake can quietly stall progress by reinforcing sugar dependence. If you select to eat them, do so in moderation and infrequently.

Fruits to Avoid

- Apples
- Apricots
- Bananas
- Cantaloupe
- Cherries
- Dates
- Dried Fruits
- Figs
- Fruit Concentrates
- Fruit Juices (all types)
- Fruit Purées
- Grapes
- Honeydew
- Kiwi
- Mango
- Nectarines
- Olive Products (containing added sugars or preservatives)
- Olives (stuffed with sweetened fillings)
- Olives (when marinated in seed oils)
- Oranges
- Papaya
- Peaches

- Pears
- Pineapple
- Plums
- Pomegranate
- Raisins
- Tangerines
- Watermelon

Vegetables to Avoid

- Acorn Squash
- Artichokes
- Beets
- Butternut Squash
- Carrots
- Cassava (Yuca)
- Corn (all varieties)
- Fingerling Potatoes
- Golden Potatoes
- Parsnips
- Peas
- Plantains
- Pumpkin
- Red Bell Pepper
- Red Potatoes

- Russet Potatoes
- Sweet Potatoes
- Taro
- Vegetable Juices
- Vegetable Purées
- White Potatoes
- Winter Squash (all varieties)
- Yams
- Yellow Potatoes

Whole Grains, Rice, and Nuts to Avoid

These grains, rice, and nuts are generally excluded due to their carbohydrate density and impact on your blood sugar. If you select to eat or use them, do so in moderation and infrequently.

Whole Grains to Avoid

- All-Purpose Flour
- Almond Flour
- Arrowroot Starch
- Baked Goods Made with Grain Flours
- Barley
- Barley Flour
- Bleached Flour
- Bread (all varieties)
- Bread Flour

- Brown Rice Flour
- Buckwheat Flour
- Cassava Flour
- Cassava Starch
- Cereals (all varieties)
- Chickpea (Garbanzo) Flour
- Coconut Flour
- Corn Flour
- Corn Starch
- Cornmeal
- Crackers (all varieties)
- Dextrin
- English Muffins (all varieties)
- Enriched Flour
- Gluten-Free Flour Blends
- Lentil Flour
- Maltodextrin
- Multigrain Bread
- Oat Flour
- Oatmeal (all varieties)
- Oats
- Pasta (all varieties)
- Potato Flour
- Potato Starch

- Rice Starch
- Rye
- Rye Flour
- Tapioca Flour
- Tapioca Starch
- Tortillas
- Unbleached Flour
- Wheat
- Wheat Flour (all types)
- Wheat Starch
- White Bread
- White Flour
- White Rice Flour
- Whole Grain Bread
- Whole Wheat Products

Rice to Avoid

- Basmati Rice
- Brown Rice
- Jasmine Rice
- Rice Blends
- White Rice
- Wild Rice

Nuts to Avoid

- Cashews
- Chestnuts
- Honey-Roasted Nuts
- Nut Butters (containing added sugars or made with seed oil)
- Nut Mixes, Flavored (containing starches or sugars)
- Nuts Roasted in Seed Oils
- Nuts, Candied Nuts
- Pistachios
- Sweetened Nuts
- Trail Mixes (containing seed oils or other unapproved ingredients)

Eggs, Milk, and Other Dairy Products to Avoid

Certain types of milk and dairy are best avoided because many are heavily processed and designed more for texture and taste than for supporting metabolic health. They may contain seed oils, added sugars, or stabilizers, and some raise your blood sugar quickly without providing lasting feelings of fullness. Even when labeled as natural or healthy, these products can quietly interfere with your metabolism, making it harder for your body to repair and regulate itself over time. If you select to eat or use them, do so in moderation and infrequently.

Eggs to Avoid

- Egg Breakfast Products (sandwiches, wraps, or bowls containing refined grains or seed oils)
- Egg Products Containing Added Sugars or Sweetened Flavorings
- Egg Products Containing Seed Oils or Vegetable Oils
- Fried Eggs Cooked in Seed Oils
- Liquid Egg Substitutes
- Packaged Egg Products Containing Preservatives or Fillers
- Pre-Cooked Egg Products Containing Preservatives or Fillers

Milks to Avoid

- Almond Milk
- Cashew Milk
- Creamers Containing Added Sugars or Seed Oils
- Creamers Shelf-Stabilized with Gums or Emulsifiers
- Flavored Milk
- Low-Fat Milk
- Oat Milk
- Reduced Fat Milk
- Rice Milk
- Skim Milk

- Soy Milk
- Sweetened Milke

Cheese to Avoid

- American Cheese
- Cheese Spread
- Fat-Free Cheese
- Flavored Cheese (with added sugars or starches)
- Low-Fat Cheese
- Nacho Cheese Sauce
- Pasteurized Cheese Food
- Processed Cheese Slices

Cottage Cheese to Avoid

- Cottage Cheese with Gum, Starches, or Stabilizers (check ingredients)
- Diet or Engineered High Protein Cottage Cheese (check ingredients)
- Flavored Cottage Cheese
- Fruit Added Cottage Cheese
- Low-Fat or Fat-Free Cottage Cheese
- Sweetened Cottage Cheese (typically found in single-serve cups)

Yogurt to Avoid

- Drinkable Yogurt
- Favored Yogurt (all varieties)

- Frozen Yogurt
- Fruit-on-the-bottom Yogurt
- Low-Fat or Fat-Free Yogurt
- Sweetened Yogurt
- Yogurt Containing Added Sugars, Syrups, or Fruit Purées
- Yogurt Containing Granola or Mix-ins
- Yogurt Containing Gums, Starches, or Thickeners
- Yogurt Containing Seed Oils

Unhealthy Oils and Fats to Avoid

Seed oils are heavily processed, unstable, and widely used in modern foods in ways the human body was never designed to handle. They promote inflammation, disrupt normal metabolism, and make it harder for your body to heal and regulate energy levels properly. Because they are hidden in many packaged and restaurant foods, they quietly undermine your health even when your overall eating habits appear reasonable.

Oils to Avoid

- Canola Oil
- Corn Oil
- Cottonseed Oil
- Grapeseed Oil
- Peanut Oil
- Rice Bran Oil
- Safflower Oil

- Seed Oil Blends
- Soybean Oil
- Sunflower Oil
- Vegetable Oil

Fats to Avoid

- Artificial Butter Substitutes and Spreads
- Butter-Flavored Oils or Sprays
- Cooking Sprays Containing Propellants and Seed Oils
- Hydrogenated Oils
- Margarine
- Partially Hydrogenated Oils
- Shelf-Stable Fats with Added Flavorings, Colors, or Preservatives
- Shortening
- Vegetable Shortening Blends

Spices, Condiments, and Sweeteners to Avoid

If you select to use any of the spices, condiments, or sweeteners listed, do so in moderation and infrequently. Some may be made healthy-eating-lifestyle-friendly when using approved ingredients.

Spices to Avoid

- Barbecue Rubs with Sugar or Honey

- Flavor Enhancers Containing MSG and/or Added Sugars
- Pre-Mixed Sauces Labeled as Spices or Seasonings
- Seasoning Packets with Added Sugars or Starches (taco, chili, etc.)
- Seasonings Containing Seed Oils
- Spice Blends Containing Maltodextrin or Dextrose
- Spice Blends with Flour-Based Fillers
- Sweetened Spice Blends

Condiments to Avoid

- Barbecue Sauce or Glaze
- Brown Mustard (made with added sugar or syrups)
- Chutneys
- Cocktail Sauce
- Condiment Blends Labeled Sauce-Style or Spread
- Duck Sauce
- Flavored Mustards (made with added sugars or syrups)
- Hoisin Sauce
- Honey Mustard
- Honey-Based Sauces and Glazes
- Ketchup
- Marinades with Added Sugars, Syrups, or Seed Oils

- Mayonnaise Made with Seed Oils
- Mustards Containing Seed Oils, Starches, or Fillers
- Pasta Sauces with Added Sugars or Seed Oils
- Relish
- Salad Dressings Containing Seed Oils or Sugars
- Sauce-Style Mustards (formulated more like dressings than seasonings)
- Steak Sauces with Added Sugars or Seed Oils
- Sweet Chili Sauce or Glaze
- Sweet Mustard (with added sugar or syrups)
- Sweet Pickles
- Sweet-and-Sour Sauce
- Tartar Sauce with Added Sugars or Seed Oils
- Teriyaki Sauce or Glaze

Sweeteners to Avoid

Refined sugars show up in far more everyday foods than most people realize, making it easy to consume much more than intended over the course of a day. That steady overexposure strains the body's ability to regulate blood sugar, increases inflammation, and contributes to insulin resistance, weight gain, and cardiovascular stress over time. If you choose to use them, do so infrequently and in moderation.

- Acesulfame Potassium (Ace-K)
- Agave Syrup
- Aspartame
- Beet Sugar

- Brown Sugar
- Cane Juice Crystals
- Cane Sugar
- Coconut Sugar
- Corn Syrup
- Date Sugar
- Date Syrup
- Evaporated Cane Juice
- Glucose Syrup
- Honey Syrup
- Honey-Flavored Products
- Honey, Blended
- Honey, Commercial (all forms)
- Honey, Locally Sourced
- Honey, Natural
- Honey, Pasteurized
- Honey, Processed Products
- Honey, Raw
- Malt Syrup
- Maltitol
- Maple Syrup
- Molasses (use only in infrequent, limited amounts; functions like other sugars)
- Powdered Confectioners' Sugar

- Rice Syrup
- Saccharin
- Sorbitol
- Sucralose
- White Sugar
- Xylitol

Key Points to Remember from Chapter 5

The following key points from Chapter 5 serve as road signs to guide your progress on your healthy eating lifestyle journey.

- Recognizing foods that consistently derail your metabolic progress is as important as choosing foods that support it.
- Foods you should avoid are not because they are unfamiliar or indulgent, but because they disrupt blood sugar regulation and cellular repair.
- Processing matters more than labels; even whole foods can become problematic when refined, sweetened, or industrially altered.
- Frequent exposure to sugars, starches, seed oils, and additives quietly undermines your metabolic stability over time.
- You maintain a healthy eating lifestyle by avoiding certain foods that are commonly accepted on other eating plans.

Chapter 6: Staying on Course

Side Roads, Rest Stops, and Knowing Your Progress

"The end of a matter is better than its beginning, and patience is better than pride." – Ecclesiastes 7:8 (NIV)

Progress on a healthy eating lifestyle is rarely uninterrupted. Changing home, work, and life schedules, eating while traveling, holiday meals, eating during special occasions, and even basic social gatherings can occasionally throw you off your eating routine. These situations are not unusual or unexpected. They are part of living in the real world and can be anticipated, accommodated, and recovered from without losing sight of the journey. You can think of them as side roads to your destination.

How you respond when these disruptions occur determines if you will continue your journey or give up and return to unhealthy eating habits. But these side roads do not need to become stopping points. Rather than viewing them as failures, think of them as temporary departures that call for better awareness of how food impacts your health, particularly how you feel mentally and physically. The good news is you can easily return to your original path.

Part of maintaining your forward progress is recognizing the foundational role of restful sleep and appropriate physical activity in sustaining a healthy eating lifestyle. You can think of them as the rest stops of the *Road Map* metaphor. Getting enough quality sleep keeps the body refreshed and supports hormonal regulation of appetite and feelings of fullness. Adequate sleep also enhances the body's ability to burn stored fat efficiently, preserve muscle mass, and recover from daily physical and metabolic stresses. Similarly, appropriate physical activity supports circulation, maintains strength, and reinforces your metabolic healing without requiring excessive time or intensity. You may not think of physical activity as a rest stop, but it helps you sleep better and make forward progress on your journey! Quality sleep and appropriate physical activity provide the rest and support the physical readiness you will find most helpful in continuing to make consistent progress on your journey.

One challenge with any eating plan is tracking progress. Modern body composition scales, or smart scales, can be used to monitor changes in weight and overall body composition over time. While these scales do not directly measure metabolism, they can provide helpful indicators of changes in fat loss, muscle maintenance, and overall progress. But having such a scale is not required in following a healthy eating lifestyle. A simple old-fashioned bathroom scale and a tape measure are really all that you need.

To help you stay oriented in tracking your progress, the *Road Map* uses two familiar dashboard readings. Body weight, recorded in pounds or kilograms, functions like a speedometer by reflecting your short-term changes and current momentum (speed of progress). Body measurements, tracked as changes in inches, centimeters, clothing sizes, or fit, function like an odometer, reflecting how your progress accumulates over time (the distance you've traveled toward your destination). Together, these simple indicators are perhaps the best ways to monitor how you are doing with your healthy eating lifestyle.

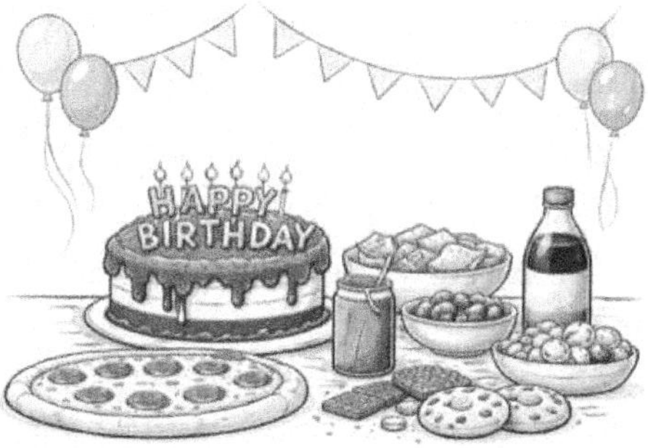

Managing Disrupted Eating Patterns

Every long journey includes side roads. Some are chosen intentionally, while others become necessary as conditions change along the way. In your healthy eating journey, disrupted eating patterns often appear as side roads taken during travel, holidays, social gatherings, periods of emotional stress, or shifts in routines. These experiences are not signs that you have left the journey; instead, they reflect real-life movement along the way. What matters most is how you prepare for these side roads and how you return to the main route afterward.

When you recognize in advance that certain events and circumstances may lead you onto a side road, you reduce their ability to disrupt your progress. Instead of reacting in the moment, you can approach these situations in advance with awareness and intention. You can decide ahead of time how flexible you will be with your food selections, identify foods that work well for you outside your routine, and remind yourself that taking a side road does not erase the distance you have already traveled.

While you are on a side road, your focus shifts from optimization to steadiness. You are not trying to accelerate progress or correct course immediately; you are simply aiming to avoid unnecessary disruption. Prioritizing protein, limiting refined carbohydrates, eating until comfortably full, and avoiding continuous snacking will help you stay oriented even when conditions are less structured. You may eat differently than usual, but you do so deliberately rather than impulsively.

Side roads are also a time to rely more on internal cues than on rigid rules. Paying attention to hunger, fullness, energy, and emotional state allows you to make reasonable choices without turning the experience into a test of willpower. When flexibility is guided and intentional, it remains supportive rather than destabilizing.

Equally important is how and when you return to the main route. The goal is not correction or compensation, but resumption. Returning simply means re-establishing your usual eating windows, prioritizing sleep, resuming gentle activity, and allowing your body to settle back into its familiar rhythm as soon as possible. The sooner you return to these practices, the shorter the impact of the side road will be.

Over time, side roads become instructive rather than discouraging. Each experience offers insight into what helps you remain steady, what feels disruptive, and what supports recovery most effectively. As this understanding grows, you approach future disruptions with greater confidence and less emotional stress.

When disrupted eating patterns are viewed through the lens of the side roads you take, they lose much of their power to discourage you. You are not off course; you are simply navigating a different stretch of the journey for a short period of time. With preparation, intentional choices, and a calm return to routine, side roads remain part of forward movement rather than obstacles to lasting progress.

Preparing in Advance for Disruptions to Healthy Eating

Preparing for disrupted eating patterns begins before you ever encounter them. When you anticipate situations that may lead you onto a side road, you place yourself in a position of calm control rather than a reactive one. One of the most effective preparations is to avoid arriving hungry. Eating a simple, protein-focused meal at home beforehand helps you enter social gatherings, travel days, or long events without the urgency that drives overeating. When hunger is already managed, you are far less likely to eat everything in sight or make choices you did not intend to make. Preparation may also include deciding in advance how flexible you will be, reminding yourself of your priorities, and accepting that the goal during these moments is steadiness, not progress.

Eating Choices During Times of Disruption

While you are on a side road, your focus shifts to making supportive choices within imperfect conditions. You are not trying to recreate your ideal routine; you are choosing the best available options. Prioritizing protein helps stabilize appetite and energy, while limiting refined carbohydrates reduces cravings and prevents escalation. Eating slowly, stopping when comfortably full, and avoiding continuous grazing help you remain oriented even when structure is limited. The aim is not restriction, but intention—choosing in a way that supports your body rather than reacting to availability, emotion, or social pressure.

Returning to Your Route After Disruptions

Returning to the main route is a matter of resumption, not repair. As soon as the disruption passes, you return to your usual eating windows, food choices, sleep habits, and gentle activity. There is no need for aggressive fasting or restrictive behavior to "undo" anything. Your body responds best to consistency, and returning calmly to familiar patterns allows your internal rhythm to re-establish itself naturally. The quicker you resume what works, the less influence the side road has on your overall progress. If you feel more comfortable thinking you need a change, reduce or eliminate carbohydrates while retaining the emphasis foremost on quality protein, accompanied by supportive healthy fats.

Over time, these strategies build confidence. Each experience teaches you that disruptions can be anticipated, navigated, and resolved without drama. You learn that progress is not defined by uninterrupted perfection, but by your ability to prepare wisely, choose intentionally, and return steadily to the route you have chosen.

Supporting Progress Through Sleep

High-quality sleep works best for you when it is treated as a consistent, intentional part of your daily rhythm rather than an afterthought. When you sleep well, your body calms, hunger signals steady, cravings soften, and emotional balance becomes easier to maintain. Sleep serves as a nightly reset that prepares you—physically and mentally—for the next day's travel on your healthy eating journey.

As your sleep becomes more consistent, your body begins to coordinate hunger, fullness, and energy more naturally. Hormones that influence appetite and stress start working in better alignment, which helps you experience fewer sudden hunger spikes and fewer misleading cravings. You may notice that mornings feel less rushed by hunger and that fasting windows begin with far less discomfort.

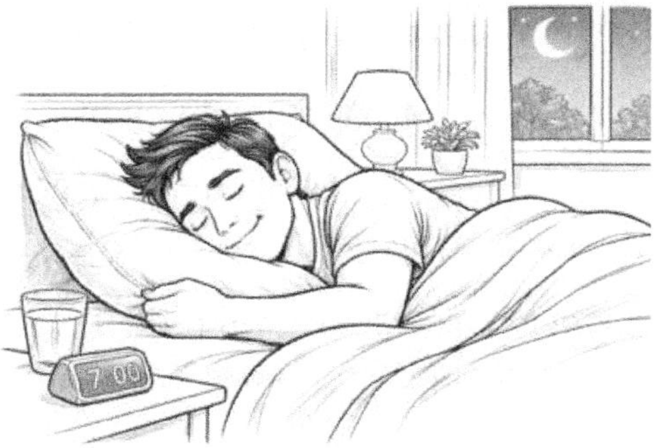

Adequate sleep also plays a vital role in reducing cravings for sugar and processed carbohydrates. When you are rested, your brain's reward system is calmer, making impulse-driven eating less likely. Emotional cravings often fade, allowing you to stay aligned with your eating principles without feeling deprived or strained.

While you sleep, your body quietly restores itself. Blood sugar regulation improves, stored energy becomes more accessible, and cells recover from daily stress. These behind-the-scenes processes support fat-burning, especially when paired with structured eating patterns such as OMAD, TMAD, intermittent fasting, or occasional alternate-day extended fasting. Over time, this strengthens your metabolic flexibility and supports steady, lasting progress.

When your sleep is inconsistent or insufficient, stress hormones rise, making fasting harder and emotional eating more tempting. By prioritizing sleep, you lower stress, stabilize your mood, and give yourself greater capacity to navigate daily choices without feeling overwhelmed or reactive.

Consistent sleep also sharpens your thinking and decision-making. When you are well rested, you tend to make clearer, more intentional choices and experience fewer moments of regret or impulse. Progress is built on small, repeated decisions, and sleep quietly strengthens your ability to make those choices well—day after day.

Practical Sleep Guidelines

- Aim for 7–9 hours of sleep each night.
- Keep your bedtime and wake time as consistent as possible from day to day.
- Establish a simple wind-down routine by dimming lights and reducing screen use.
- Avoid eating several hours before bed, so your sleep isn't dominated by digestion.
- Think of sleep as a metabolic tool that supports fat-burning, appetite control, and emotional steadiness.

Supporting Progress Through Physical Activity

Like sleep, physical activity works best for you when it is simple, consistent, and free from pressure. Your goal is not to train hard or push your limits, but to maintain your muscle tone as you move forward on your healthy eating journey. Gentle movement supports your circulation, protects muscle, and reinforces metabolic stability without adding stress, making it a natural companion to dietary change.

As your body adapts to weight loss and reduced carbohydrate intake, it may attempt to conserve energy by reducing muscle mass. This is where gentle, regular movement becomes especially important for you. By remaining lightly active, you signal to your body that muscle is still needed, helping you preserve strength, mobility, and metabolic rate so that fat—not muscle—is lost during the healing process.

As muscle is preserved, your body becomes more efficient at using energy. Movement improves blood flow and supports cellular efficiency, helping you maintain a calmer internal environment. This steadiness supports fasting and low-carbohydrate eating with less resistance, allowing your daily routines to feel more manageable rather than draining.

In addition to its physical benefits, gentle activity helps you reduce emotional and habitual triggers around eating. Simple movement gives you a healthy outlet for stress, lowering the likelihood that you will eat in response to emotion rather than hunger. As movement becomes routine for you, older carbohydrate-driven patterns gradually begin to lose their influence.

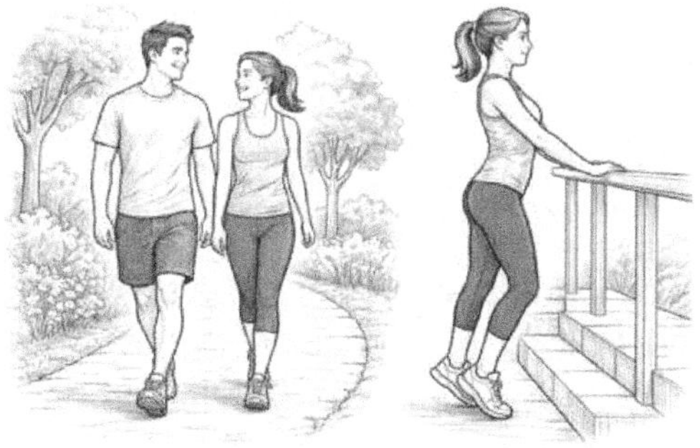

Light activity, such as slow walking, stretching, or basic mobility work, can also help you maintain fasting windows. Improved circulation and reduced stiffness help prevent feelings of lethargy, particularly during OMAD or TMAD eating patterns. Many people notice that when they stay gently active, fasting feels more natural and requires less effort.

Over time, regular movement reinforces discipline and steadiness while supporting the healthier identity you are building. Each small session reminds you that progress is maintained through consistency rather than intensity. In this way, activity supports your emotional resilience, physical comfort, and long-term sustainability—key elements for staying on course along the *Road Map.*

Practical Activity Guidelines

- Aim for 45–90 minutes of gentle movement per week, not per day.
- Break activities into small sessions, as brief as 5–10 minutes each.
- Choose comfortable, accessible movements such as leisurely walking, stretching, light range-of-motion routines, or household movement.
- Understand that lifting weights is an option, but is not required. Isometric exercises (where you use your own body weight to strengthen yourself) can be done at home without joining a gym or buying expensive exercise equipment.
- Focus on consistency rather than intensity in your activity choices, especially if you are heavier. Reintroduce movement carefully, managing joint or flexibility concerns as you do so.
- Treat physical activity as a supportive tool for preserving muscle, improving circulation, and maintaining emotional stability, not as a necessary evil.
- Choose physical activities you like and would prefer doing rather than those selected for you by others, unless suggested or required by a health care practitioner.

Sleeping and activity work together to keep your journey steady. Sleep restores balance each night, preparing your body and mind for the day ahead. At the same time, gentle activity keeps your body capable, preserves muscle, and supports metabolic stability as you move forward. When practiced consistently and without pressure, these two habits create a reliable rhythm that supports healing, strengthens daily decision-making, and helps you remain on course. Together, sleeping and activity provide the foundation that allows progress to unfold naturally as you continue along the *Road Map* toward better health.

Monitoring Progress Over Time

As you continue following the *Road Map,* progress is best understood through indicators rather than expectations. Just as a vehicle provides feedback through its dashboard, your healthy eating journey offers signals that help you understand your progress. Two of the most helpful indicators in this metaphor are the speedometer (weight) and the odometer (measurements).

The speedometer reflects your body weight and how you're responding to the healthy eating journey right now. When your speed is appropriate, weight changes tend to be gradual rather than erratic, and your daily routines feel steady rather than strained. You notice positive impacts on your daily energy, hunger intensity, sleep quality, mood stability, and mental clarity. Hunger is present but manageable, fasting windows feel reasonable, and cravings are quieter. These indicators suggest you are moving at a sustainable pace.

When the speedometer indicates that you may be moving too fast (losing weight too quickly), warning signs often appear. You might notice persistent fatigue, disrupted sleep, increased irritability, heightened cravings, or abrupt, unstable weight changes. These signals do not mean failure; they indicate that your pace may need adjustment. Slowing weight loss slightly by easing fasting windows and changing foods you eat can help restore balance to how fast your weight is being reduced without the adverse side effects.

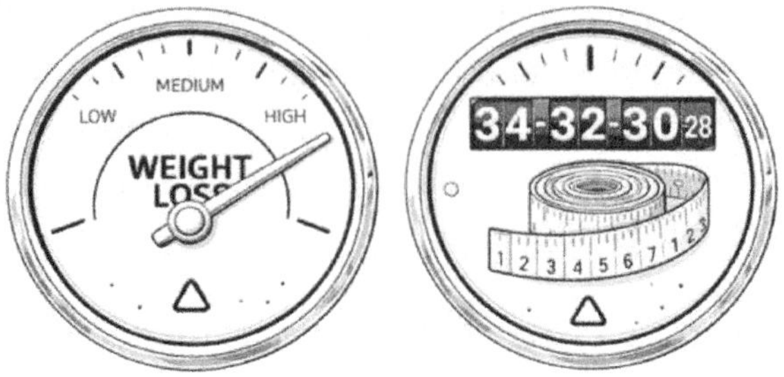

The odometer, by contrast, reflects distance traveled over time. It represents the cumulative progress you have made, measured by physical measurements rather than day-to-day weight changes. Odometer indicators include inches or centimeters lost at the waist, hips, or other areas; improved clothing fit; reductions in belt size; increased ease of movement; and improved health markers in your blood work. These measurements confirm that forward movement is occurring even when your weight speedometer values appear unchanged.

Used together, the speedometer and odometer help you avoid two common mistakes. Focusing only on weight can lead to impatience or unnecessary course corrections. Focusing only on measurements can cause you to ignore early warning signs that your pace may be unsustainable. When you pay attention to both, you gain a more accurate and balanced understanding of where you are on the journey.

Monitoring progress in this way keeps your focus grounded and realistic. You are not chasing perfection or forcing outcomes. Instead, you are learning to read your body's feedback, adjust your pace wisely, and trust that steady movement adds up. The speedometer keeps you attentive to the present moment, while the odometer reassures you that the journey is unfolding—even when progress feels gradual.

Key Points to Remember from Chapter 6

The following key points from Chapter 6 serve as road signs to guide your progress on your healthy eating lifestyle journey.

- Sleeping and activity work together as a foundation for steady, sustainable progress.
- Consistent sleep serves as a daily reset, helping regulate hunger, cravings, stress, and decision-making, making healthy eating patterns easier to maintain.
- Gentle, low-pressure physical activity preserves muscle, supports circulation, and stabilizes metabolism without adding unnecessary strain on your body.
- Progress is best monitored using both the speedometer (weight) to observe short-term trends and the odometer (measurements) to recognize long-term progress.
- Disrupted eating patterns are best understood as side roads taken, not failures in your eating patterns, and can be navigated successfully through preparation, intentional choices during those side road events, and a calm return to established routines.
- Lasting progress is built through consistency, awareness, and the ability to remain oriented toward the destination even when the journey includes side roads.

Chapter 7: Starting Your Journey

Entering the On-Ramp

"Therefore, since we are surrounded by such a great cloud of witnesses, let us throw off everything that hinders and the sin that so easily entangles. And let us run with perseverance the race marked out for us." – Hebrews 12:1 (NIV)

You are now at the point where your understanding of the *Road Map to a Healthy Eating Lifestyle* can be turned into action. Rather than asking you to change everything at once, this healthy eating schedule provides a measured entry into the *Road Map* through a series of intentional weekly steps. The schedule begins by focusing on food quality and daily timing, then gradually introduces eating windows and fasting patterns.

The purpose of the schedule is not to force progress, but to help you develop sustainable habits that make healthy eating a natural, repeatable part of everyday life. You are free to make modifications to it as your progress dictates. As mentioned throughout the *Road Map,* if you run into any difficulties in adopting any eating practice, be sure to stop doing it. And be sure to keep your primary care physician informed of your progress and any issues you encounter along the way.

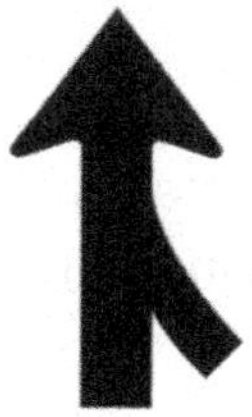

Week 1: Establishing the Foundation

Focus: Choosing Quality Food and Creating Daily Rhythms

- Eliminate all seed oils from your cooking, packaged foods, and condiments.
- Follow the Foods to Eat and Foods to Avoid guidelines consistently.
- Stop eating at least 3 hours before your bedtime.
- Delay your first meal until 90 minutes after waking.
- Use a 12-hour eating window, adjusted earlier or later based on your daily schedule.
- Eat two or three meals within the window, avoiding snacking.

Week 2: Introducing Time-Restricted Eating

Focus: Adding a 12 to 14-Hour Fasting Window

- Establish a 12 to 14-hour fasting window that includes your overnight sleeping time.
- Set eating windows such as 8 a.m. to 8 p.m. or 10 a.m. to 8 p.m., with slightly varying start times across the week.
- Maintain your food quality and protein prioritization.
- Reduce your meals to two or three, based on your hunger cues.
- Optionally introduce apple cider vinegar with the mother, diluted in water, added to your cooking, or taken as a capsule in the morning and before bedtime.

- Optionally introduce olive oil, taken with water, added to your cooking, or taken as a softgel in the morning and before bedtime.
- Optionally introduce omegas 3, 6, and 9 with turmeric, taken as a softgel in the morning and before bedtime.

Week 3: Strengthening the Fasting Pattern

Focus: Extending the Fasting Window to 14 to 16 Hours

- Extend your fasting window to 14-16 hours.
- Use eating windows such as 11 a.m. to 7 p.m. or 12 p.m. to 8 p.m., alternating days.
- Begin consolidating your meals into two meals per day as hunger allows.
- Monitor your energy, sleep quality, and recovery.

Week 4: Targeting an Intermittent Fasting Range

Focus: Extending the Fasting Window to 16 to 18 Hours

- Extend your fasting window to 16-18 hours.
- Use eating windows such as 1 p.m.to 7 p.m. or 2 p.m. to 8 p.m., rotating as needed.
- Establish TMAD (two meals a day) as your default eating pattern.
- Avoid increasing your portion sizes to make up for fasting.

Week 5: Stabilization and Pattern Awareness

Focus: Varying Your Eating Patterns to Avoid Stagnating Your Progress

- Maintain your established fasting window.
- Vary eating windows by one to two hours across the week.
- Observe your hunger signals, sleep, training response, and mental clarity.
- Adjust your food composition (focus on protein) before altering your fasting duration.

Week 6: Introducing Alternate Day Fasting

Focus: Adding Full Days of Total Fasting

- Add two alternate fasting days to your week, separated by at least one eating day.
- Consume water, electrolytes, and non-caloric beverages on your fasting day(s).
- Resume normal Road Map eating the day following a fast without eating extra food.
- Maintain variable eating windows on your eating days.

Week 7: TMAD as the Standard, OMAD as an Option

Focus: Exploring Eating Options

- Use Two Meals a Day (TMAD) as your primary daily eating routine.

- Try One Meal a Day (OMAD) if you would like to experiment with a different eating routine.
- Align your meal frequency with your activity level, stress, and recovery needs.

Week 8: Staying on Course

Focus: Looking Ahead to the Rest of Your Journey

- Periodically evaluate your progress and determine whether changes are needed.
- Stay aware of recent developments in maintaining a healthy eating lifestyle.
- Keep track of your progress to be alert to how foods and eating patterns impact your journey.

Chapter 8: Enjoying Your Destination

Maintaining Your Success

"Let us not become weary in doing good, for at the proper time we will reap a harvest if we do not give up."
– Galatians 6:9 (NIV)

Maintaining the results you have achieved begins with continuing to use the *Road Map* as a point of reference rather than viewing it as something you have completed and set aside. Throughout your journey, you have learned to orient yourself by clear principles and practices, and they remain the foundation for living well and maintaining your success.

As you remain attentive to these principles and practices, you continue to benefit from being consciously aware of how and when you eat. Allowing space between meals, being intentional about eating windows, and keeping carbohydrates in proper proportion to protein are not temporary strategies. Together, they establish patterns that support a healthy metabolism. Living out these principles and practices is no longer about reaching a destination, but about sustaining health over time.

This same mindset now extends to how you manage sleep, activity, and the inevitable disruptions of daily life. Prioritizing rest and maintaining regular movement supports recovery, balance, and long-term resilience. Preparing for travel, celebrations, and unexpected detours allows you to navigate them without losing direction. By continuing to apply what you have learned across these areas, you care for the whole journey, not just the meals along the way.

Making Wise Food Choices

Knowing which foods to eat and which to avoid remains central to your long-term relationship with food. You have seen how food quality influences energy and recovery. Continuing to choose whole, minimally processed foods allows you to maintain your results. At this point in your journey, you can now experiment with adding back into your healthy eating plan some—not all—of the foods that were identified as ones to avoid. These foods contain ingredients that would gradually undermine your progress on the journey. But now you must consider how adding some of them back into your eating plans could negate the progress you have made. The best practice, of course, would be to avoid them entirely, but some of the foods to avoid have probably been on your lifelong favorites list. If you choose to add some of the foods back into your eating plan, you will want to limit how much you eat and how often you eat them. Since some of the foods to avoid are higher in sugar, it is essential to remember that sugar raises insulin levels, which, over time, can promote fat storage and weight gain.

Using Fasting for Ongoing Maintenance

Fasting, when used wisely, remains a practical tool for tuning your metabolic engine. When eating patterns drift, or you feel you are slipping back into old habits, fasting provides a structured way to reset appetite signals, restore metabolic flexibility, and reestablish rhythm without abandoning the principles you have already learned.

Fasting supports your body's natural internal maintenance processes. During periods without food, the body shifts attention from constant digestion to cellular repair and renewal. This includes removing damaged or inefficient cells and recycling their components to support healthier function going forward. Even at your destination, this process continues. The occasional fast can reinforce your body's efforts in ongoing cellular repair and help you maintain your healthy eating lifestyle.

Navigating Detours and Disruptions

Planning for disruptions to eating healthy meals is now a familiar part of your experience on the *Road Map*. You have come to recognize that travel, holidays, social gatherings, and unexpected schedule changes will happen. But rather than viewing these moments as failures or setbacks, you now approach them with preparation, awareness, and realistic expectations.

On your journey, you will have learned how your body responds to various types of food, allowing you to make thoughtful choices of the foods you eat during times of disruption. You now know when disruptions are on the horizon so that you can prepare in advance. When disruptions are unexpected, you know to choose wisely and limit your food choices to be compatible with your healthy eating lifestyle. Disruptions do not remove you from the journey; they alter the scenery for a time. With experience, you have learned to rejoin the main route smoothly, carrying forward what works rather than starting over. This perspective allows you to live fully while maintaining progress, reinforcing that a healthy eating lifestyle is flexible, resilient, and sustainable over the long term.

Maintaining Health with Sleep and Activity

Sleep and activity continue to serve as essential roles as you maintain your progress. Throughout your journey, they supported your progress, and now they help you preserve it. By maintaining consistent rest and regular movement, you support your body's natural processes of repair and muscle retention, creating the conditions that support lasting metabolic health.

Adequate sleep allows your body to continue repairing, regulating hormones, and managing stress, all of which influence appetite, energy, and long-term metabolic health. When sleep is consistently compromised, even well-established eating habits can become harder to sustain. You have learned that prioritizing rest supports clearer thinking, steadier energy, and better decision-making. Protecting your sleep schedule whenever possible helps keep your healthy eating lifestyle predictable and manageable.

Activity serves a similar role in maintaining your success. You are no longer exercising to compensate for eating or to chase performance goals. Instead, regular movement supports circulation, muscle preservation, insulin sensitivity, and overall resilience. Simple, repeatable activities, such as walking and light isometric exercises, help keep your body strong and capable without adding unnecessary strain.

Together, sleep and activity reinforce the body's natural processes of repair and renewal. Consistent rest and regular movement support tissue maintenance, metabolic balance, and hormonal regulation, helping your body continue functioning well over time. By giving attention to both sleep and activity, you create the conditions that allow these processes to reinforce your healthy eating lifestyle and support long-term success.

Revisiting the Key Points to Remember

An essential part of maintaining your progress is periodically revisiting the Key Points to Remember at the end of each chapter. These summaries function as dependable mile markers you can consult whenever a quick refresher of key principles and practices is needed. Reviewing them in mind can prevent gradual drift back into old habits and allow you to make early course corrections when needed. You are not returning to the Key Points to relearn the journey, but to reaffirm what you have found to be effective for you.

In support of the material in the *Road Map* and the Key Points to Remember, the “Roadside Assistance” chapter extends this support by providing resources you can return to as needed, helping you continue to develop and maintain this lifestyle as your journey unfolds.

Keep pressing on and building upon your success!

Key Points to Remember from Chapter 8

The following key points from Chapter 8 serve as road signs to guide your progress on your healthy eating lifestyle journey.

- Living at the destination means continuing to use the *Road Map* as a trusted reference, not something you leave behind once progress has been made.
- The principles and practices you learned along the journey remain the foundation for maintaining your success and supporting long-term health.

- Wise food choices continue to matter, even as flexibility increases. Quality, proportion, and frequency protect the progress you have achieved.
- Fasting remains a supportive tool you can use intentionally to recalibrate eating patterns and reinforce metabolic health when needed.
- Sleep and activity sustain the body's natural processes of repair and muscle retention, creating the conditions that support lasting metabolic health.
- Disruptions such as travel, celebrations, and schedule changes are expected parts of life and can be navigated without losing direction.
- Revisiting the Key Points to Remember from earlier chapters helps keep healthy eating principles and practices fresh and prevents gradual drift.

Chapter 9: Roadside Assistance

Consulting Reliable Resources

"Now the Bereans were of more noble character than the Thessalonians, for they received the message with great eagerness and examined the Scriptures every day to see if what Paul said was true." – Acts 17:11 (NIV)

Chapter 8 serves as the closing section of this *Road Map* and is intentionally designed as a place you can return to over time. Central to this section is the companion website, which serves as the primary hub for ongoing updates, expanded resources, and future additions related to healthy eating and metabolic health:

https://edcot.info/healthy-eating

This website is intended to remain a living extension of the *Road Map,* allowing you to explore new material and stay informed about research, insights, and practical tools that continue to develop.

Articles of Interest

Additional articles are available on the companion website.

7-Day Carnivore Diet Meal Plan for Beginners, by a Dietitian
https://thenutritioninsider.com/learn/carnivore-diet-meal-plan-for-beginners/

Carnivore Diet Meal Plan: Breakfast, Lunch, & Dinner
https://www.cookunity.com/blog/carnivore-diet-meal-plan

Carnivore Diet: Meal Plan, Food List, and What You Should Know
https://www.webmd.com/diet/carnivore-diet

Keto Diet Food List – Eating Well
https://www.eatingwell.com/article/291245/complete-keto-diet-food-list-what-you-can-and-cannot-eat-if-youre-on-a-ketogenic-diet/

Ketogenic Diet and Recipes
https://www.bbcgoodfood.com/recipes/collection/ketogenic-diet-recipes

Ketovore Diet and Meal Plans
https://www.gocarnivore.com/post/ketovore-diet

Ketovore Recipes
https://oliviawyles.com/ketovore-recipes

Relevant Websites

Additional websites and updated webpage links are available on the companion website.

Carnivore Diet
https://carnivore.diet/

Fasting Method
https://www.thefastingmethod.com

Go Carnivore
https://www.gocarnivore.com/

How to Carnivore
https://www.howtocarnivore.com

Keto Kamp
https://www.ketokamp.com/

Ketovore
https://ketogenic.com/what-is-ketovore-and-how-does-it-compare-to-keto/

Recommended Trip Advisors

Additional health coaches and advisors and updated links are available on the companion website.

Road Map to a Healthy Eating Lifestyle draws on the author's real-life experiences and the healthy eating and lifestyle principles of several influential practitioners, listed here in alphabetical order. There are many other excellent health advisor videos available on YouTube, but for me, these individuals have been the most helpful and consistent in creating this *Road Map,* and I have personally seen healthy results.

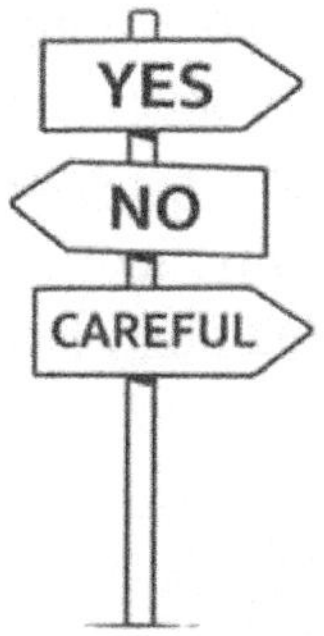

Please be aware that many of these advisors endorse a variety of products and supplements to support their YouTube channels. *As always, if you choose to take any of those supplements, be sure to check with your primary care physician first to make sure it's okay for you to take them!*

Ben Azadi – Ben's perspective emphasizes achieving metabolic freedom through keto-aligned eating principles and lifestyle strategies that support metabolic efficiency. His insights include eliminating industrial seed oils to reduce inflammation, stabilizing insulin by avoiding ultra-processed carbohydrates, and improving fat-burning capacity. He also teaches the daily use of raw apple cider vinegar with the mother and high-quality extra virgin olive oil to support digestion, insulin sensitivity, and lipid balance. Furthermore, he emphasizes strategic fasting practices, including One Meal a Day (OMAD) and Two Meals a Day (TMAD) eating windows, which help extend periods of low insulin, promote autophagy (the body's natural process of cleaning out damaged cells), support metabolic flexibility, and enhance the body's ability to utilize stored fat as fuel.

Website: www.benazadi.com

YouTube: www.youtube.com/@KetoKamp

Dr. Eric Berg, D.C. – Dr. Berg is an established health educator, author, and the founder of the Berg Institute of Health & Wellness. Drawing on more than three decades of experience in chiropractic practice and natural health, he has guided a global audience toward greater personal health awareness through clear education, evidence-based nutritional guidance, and his early leadership in healthy keto and intermittent fasting.

Website: www.drberg.com

YouTube: www.youtube.com/@Drberg

Dr. Ken D. Berry, M.D. – Dr. Berry is a board-certified family physician, and his Proper Human Diet (PHD) serves as a practical guide for restoring health. With more than two decades of experience in family medicine, I have worked with thousands of patients by applying clear, research-informed guidance shaped by longstanding ancestral principles. This approach avoids unnecessary complexity and focuses on direct, usable strategies. It emphasizes low-carbohydrate ketogenic and carnivore eating patterns, along with lifestyle practices such as intermittent and alternate day fasting, to address conditions including diabetes, obesity, hormonal imbalance, and related metabolic concerns.

Website: www.drberry.com

YouTube: www.youtube.com/@KenDBerryMD

Dr. Robert Cywes, M.D., Ph.D. – Dr. Cywes' approach focuses on carbohydrate addiction, emotional eating patterns, and reducing dependency on processed carbohydrates as a pathway to long-term metabolic improvement. His insights also include carnivore eating principles, particularly the effectiveness of animal-based nutrition in reducing hunger, stabilizing metabolic signals, limiting addictive carbohydrate triggers, and supporting nutritional simplicity for individuals seeking to overcome carbohydrate-driven behaviors.

Website: www.facebook.com/carbaddictiondoc

YouTube: www.youtube.com/@DrCywesCarbAddictionDoc

Thomas DeLauer – Thomas DeLauer is widely recognized for guiding highly occupied individuals toward meaningful improvements in health through manageable adjustments to diet and daily habits. His work focuses on helping people achieve better health while also enhancing performance in their professional and personal pursuits. The content he provides is designed to equip individuals with practical, accessible information that supports positive change without requiring the abandonment of familiar or enjoyable aspects of life.

With a career rooted in healthcare, Thomas brings extensive experience, supported by a dedicated research team that grounds recommendations in scientific evidence. This ensures that the guidance offered is both credible and compelling. At its core, this work is intended to empower individuals to perform at a higher level, reflecting the conviction that improved personal performance contributes to broader positive outcomes.

Website: www.thomasdelauer.com

YouTube: www.youtube.com/@ThomasDeLauerOfficial

Dr. Becky Gillaspy, D.C. – Dr. Gillaspy is the author of the *Intermittent Fasting Diet Guide and Cookbook.* Raised in central Pennsylvania, she graduated summa cum laude with research honors from Palmer College of Chiropractic in 1991. Her early career included years in private clinical practice and work as an on-air health consultant for a local ABC television affiliate.

Following the birth of her daughter, Dr. Becky transitioned into higher education, where she devoted the remainder of her more than 24-year professional career to teaching college-level anatomy and nutrition courses. During this time, she also earned certification as a health and wellness coach. She now focuses full-time on helping individuals achieve sustainable health and weight-management goals through her educational website and YouTube channel.

Website: https://drbeckyfitness.com

YouTube: https://www.youtube.com/@beckygillaspy

Dr. Tony Hampton – Dr. Hampton is a family and obesity medicine physician who has treated patients with complex chronic conditions since 1998. He is board-certified in Family Medicine and Obesity Medicine, holds a master's degree in Nutrition and Functional Medicine, and is a founding board member of the American Diabetes Society. His professional service also includes several board roles with health organizations. Diabetes has shaped his work on both a personal and professional level, motivating him to author, *Fix Your Diet, Fix Your Diabetes*. His educational efforts focus on diet-centered strategies for metabolic health, informed by clinical experience and ongoing engagement with nutrition-focused professional organizations.

YouTube: http://www.youtube.com/@DrTonyHampton

Dr. Livingood, D.C. – Dr. Livingood (his given name) is a Doctor of Natural Medicine, a Doctor of Chiropractic, and an Amazon best-selling author. He is the founder of Livingood Daily, an organization dedicated to helping individuals pursue practical and lasting approaches to improved health and well-being. His work focuses on identifying realistic, sustainable solutions that support daily progress toward healthier living.

His commitment to this path began in 2007 following a critical health crisis involving his father. After conventional medical approaches failed to produce meaningful improvement, Dr. Livingood pursued alternative, research-informed strategies that ultimately enabled his father to discontinue numerous medications and experience significant recovery from severe cardiac and autoimmune conditions. Building on this experience, Dr. Livingood, alongside his wife, registered nurse Jessica Livingood, and their team, provides clear, science-supported lifestyle guidance to help individuals improve how they feel, function, and live, regardless of where they are on their health journey.

Website: www.facebook.com/drlivingood

YouTube: www.youtube.com/@DrLivingood

Legend of Key Terms

The following legend of key terms serves as the Glossary for the *Road Map*. Just as a traveler must understand the symbols and markings on a map to be able to follow a route, you will benefit from understanding the following terms used throughout this journey, especially as health advisors and medical professionals frequently use them.

LEGEND

Route

Detour

On Ramp

Adaptation – the body's gradual adjustment to changes in eating patterns, fasting duration, or food choices. Adaptation explains why progress may slow and why variation can be beneficial.

Alternate Day Fasting – a structured fasting approach in which you alternate between days of eating and days of fasting. On eating days, food intake occurs within a defined eating window, whereas on fasting days, caloric intake is minimal. This pattern reduces overall insulin exposure, encourages fat burning, and supports the development of metabolic flexibility over time.

Autophagy – a natural cellular recycling process activated during fasting, in which damaged or dysfunctional cells are broken down and reused for repair and renewal.

Carnivore Eating – an eating approach centered on animal-based foods, typically excluding plant foods. This approach emphasizes protein and fat while minimizing carbohydrates to support metabolic healing and appetite regulation.

Carbohydrates (Carbs) – sugars and starches that raise blood glucose levels. While not essential for survival, carbohydrates strongly influence insulin response and metabolic state.

Consistency – regular adherence to core principles over time. Consistency, rather than intensity, drives sustainable results.

Cortisol – a hormone produced by the adrenal glands that plays a central role in the body's stress response, energy regulation, and blood sugar balance. Cortisol levels naturally follow a daily rhythm, rising in the morning and tapering throughout the day. Chronic stress, inadequate sleep, or metabolic strain can disrupt this rhythm, potentially affecting appetite, fat storage, and overall progress in a healthy eating lifestyle.

Dietary Fat – a primary energy source in low-carbohydrate eating. Fat supports satiety, hormone production, and sustained energy when carbohydrates are restricted.

Eating Window – the daily time frame during which food is consumed. Eating windows influence insulin exposure, digestion, and metabolic recovery.

Farm-Raised – a general term indicating that animals or fish are raised as part of an agricultural operation, such as pens, or an aquaculture system, such as tanks. This term does not specify living conditions, feed or water conditions, farming practices, or free access to outdoor environments, and may include confinement-based systems.

Ghrelin – a hormone produced primarily in the stomach that signals hunger to the brain; levels typically rise before meals and fall after eating. During dietary changes, especially reduced carbohydrate intake or fasting, this hormone signaling may temporarily increase as the body adjusts to new eating patterns.

GLP-1 Medications – a class of prescription medications that mimic or enhance the action of glucagon-like peptide-1 (GLP-1), a hormone involved in appetite regulation, insulin secretion, and blood glucose control. GLP-1 medications slow gastric emptying, increase feelings of fullness, and reduce appetite, which can support weight loss and improved metabolic markers. While effective for appetite modulation and short-term weight reduction, these medications do not, by themselves, establish food quality discrimination, eating patterns, or lifestyle habits required for long-term metabolic health and weight maintenance.

Insulin – a hormone that regulates blood sugar by directing glucose into cells for use or storage. Chronically elevated insulin levels hinder fat burning, contributing to weight gain and metabolic dysfunction.

Insulin Resistance – a condition in which cells respond poorly to insulin, requiring higher levels to manage blood sugar. This state often precedes weight gain, type 2 diabetes, and difficulty losing fat.

Intermittent Fasting – a structured approach to alternating periods of eating and fasting to support insulin regulation, fat burning, and metabolic flexibility.

Keto Flu – a short-term collection of symptoms that may occur during the early stages of carbohydrate reduction or ketogenic eating. Common experiences include fatigue, headache, irritability, and lightheadedness. Keto flu reflects the body's metabolic transition from primarily relying on carbohydrates to using fat and ketones for energy, and typically resolves as adaptation occurs.

Ketogenic (Keto) Eating – an eating approach that significantly restricts carbohydrates, emphasizes adequate protein, and includes healthy fats to promote ketosis and improved metabolic function.

Ketones – energy molecules produced from fat when carbohydrate intake is low. Ketones provide an alternative fuel source for the brain and body during ketosis or fasting.

Ketosis – a metabolic state in which the body primarily burns fat for fuel and produces ketones as an energy source due to low carbohydrate intake.

Ketovore – a dietary approach that combines elements of a ketogenic diet with a predominantly carnivore-based way of eating. It emphasizes animal-based foods—such as meat, eggs, and animal fats—while allowing limited amounts of low-carbohydrate, low-toxicity plant foods. The primary goal of a ketovore approach is to maintain nutritional ketosis, support metabolic health, and minimize carbohydrate intake, while offering slightly more flexibility than a strict ketogenic or carnivore diet.

Maintenance – the ongoing practice of sustaining metabolic health and eating habits after initial goals are achieved. Maintenance emphasizes awareness, flexibility, and long-term stewardship.

Metabolic Flexibility – the capacity of the body to switch between burning glucose and burning fat for fuel. Improved metabolic flexibility allows for more extended periods without food and reduces dependence on frequent carbohydrate intake.

Metabolic Freedom – a practical state in which food no longer controls appetite, energy, or decision making. Hunger becomes predictable, eating becomes intentional, and fasting becomes manageable rather than stressful.

Metabolic Health – the body's ability to efficiently regulate blood sugar, insulin, energy storage, and fat utilization. Good metabolic health supports stable energy, reduced inflammation, and long-term weight management.

Mitochondria – the structures within your cells responsible for producing energy. They convert the food you eat into usable fuel that powers movement, bodily functions, and overall metabolic activity. Because cells respond directly to the components found in food, not just calorie counts or marketing claims, the quality and processing of what you eat can either support or disrupt mitochondrial function. Foods that appear healthy on the surface may still interfere with this process at the cellular level. When mitochondria are well supported, energy production is steady and efficient; when they are disrupted, fatigue and stalled metabolic progress can occur even when calorie intake seems appropriate.

Net Carbohydrates (Net Carbs) – the total carbohydrates in a food minus the fiber, and in some cases, certain sugar alcohols. Because fiber and some sugar alcohols are not fully absorbed, net carbs are often used in low-carbohydrate eating better to estimate a food's impact on blood sugar.

OMAD (One Meal a Day) – an eating pattern in which all daily food intake occurs in a single meal, typically within a one-hour window.

Organic Food – food produced according to certified organic standards that prohibit the use of synthetic pesticides, herbicides, genetically modified organisms, antibiotics, and growth hormones. Organic food emphasizes natural growing practices, animal welfare, and minimal chemical intervention, supporting both environmental stewardship and metabolic health.

Pasteurized / Ultra Pasteurized – a food safety process in which food, most commonly dairy, is heated to reduce harmful bacteria and extend shelf life. Standard pasteurization uses lower temperatures for shorter periods and preserves more of the food's natural structure, while ultra-pasteurization uses higher temperatures to prolong shelf life significantly. Higher heat processing can further alter proteins and enzymes, which may affect texture, flavor, and how some individuals tolerate the food.

Pasture-Raised – a farming method in which land-based animals are raised primarily outdoors with regular access to pasture and natural foraging. Pasture-raised practices support more natural animal behavior, improved nutrient profiles, and alignment with whole food principles.

Processed Foods – foods altered from their natural state through industrial processing, often containing refined sugars, seed oils, and additives that disrupt metabolic health.

Protein – an essential macronutrient required for muscle maintenance, repair, immune function, and metabolic health. Adequate protein intake is foundational across all eating approaches in this *Road Map*.

Satiety – the sense of being comfortably full and satisfied after eating, rather than having stopped eating. It reflects your body's internal signal that it has received sufficient nourishment and no longer requires additional food at that time. Learning to recognize satiety is an integral part of following this *Road Map*, as it helps distinguish proper nourishment from eating driven by habit, emotion, or external cues.

Seed Oils – industrially processed vegetable oils high in omega-6 fatty acids. Excessive consumption is commonly associated with inflammation and metabolic disruption.

Subcutaneous Fat – fat stored just beneath the skin. It is the type of fat most visible on the body and is commonly associated with appearance and body shape. While subcutaneous fat contributes to overall body weight, it is generally less metabolically active than visceral fat and is often reduced later in the healthy eating journey.

TMAD (Two Meals a Day) – an eating pattern involving two meals within a defined eating window, often used as a transitional or long-term strategy. Sometimes abbreviated also as 2MAD.

Visceral Fat – fat stored deep within the abdominal cavity, surrounding internal organs such as the liver, pancreas, and intestines. This type of fat is metabolically active and closely associated with insulin resistance, inflammation, and increased risk of chronic disease. Reducing visceral fat is a primary health goal of this *Road Map*, as improvements in metabolic health often begin internally before visible changes occur.

Whole Foods – foods that remain close to their natural form, typically without added sugars, industrial oils, or artificial ingredients.

Wild-Caught (Fresh Caught) – fish harvested from their natural environment rather than raised in controlled farming systems. Wild-caught fish typically have a more natural diet, higher amounts of omega-3 fatty acids, and fewer concerns related to feed composition or confinement.

Biblical Principles for a Healthy Lifestyle

The Old Testament and New Testament together provide a kind of "road map" for bodily stewardship, beginning with God's original provision of plant-based foods in Eden, then moving through the post-Fall and post-flood expansion of diet to include meat, followed by covenant-era food boundaries under the Law that shaped Israel's practices for holiness and communal health. Along the way, Proverbs adds practical roadside warnings against gluttony, excess, and unrestrained appetite, emphasizing self-control and the real-life consequences that follow overeating and indulgence. Daniel's account then functions like a cautionary detour sign, contrasting the effects of rich royal food with the benefits of disciplined simplicity. In the New Testament, believers are taught that foods are not to be treated as spiritually defiling in themselves, and that eating is to be received with gratitude, guided by love, and limited voluntarily when a choice would wound a fellow diner's conscience. The road map culminates in the Bible's vision of restored life in the New Jerusalem, where God's provision is portrayed through the tree of life and its fruit, echoing Eden's original goodness and pointing to a final destination marked by wholeness. Below are two categories of passages to consider exploring on these biblical principles and practices.

Healthy Eating and Food Choices

Genesis 1:29 (NIV) – *"Then God said, "I give you every seed-bearing plant on the face of the whole earth and every tree that has fruit with seed in it. They will be yours for food."*

Leviticus 11:1–47 (NIV) – *A list of the clean and unclean foods under Old Testament Law*

Deuteronomy 8:7-10 (NIV) – *"For the Lord your God is bringing you into a good land—a land with brooks, streams, and deep springs gushing out into the valleys and hills; a land with wheat and barley, vines and fig trees, pomegranates, olive oil and honey; a land where bread will not be scarce and you will lack nothing; a land where the rocks are iron and you can dig copper out of the hills."*

"When you have eaten and are satisfied, praise the Lord your God for the good land he has given you."

Psalm 104:14–15 (NIV) – *"He makes grass grow for the cattle, and plants for people to cultivate—bringing forth food from the earth: wine that gladdens human hearts, oil to make their faces shine, and bread that sustains their hearts."*

Proverbs 23:20–21 (NIV) – *"Do not join those who drink too much wine or gorge themselves on meat, for drunkards and gluttons become poor, and drowsiness clothes them in rags."*

Proverbs 25:16 (NIV) – *"If you find honey, eat just enough—too much of it, and you will vomit."*

Isaiah 55:2 (NIV) – *"Why spend money on what is not bread, and your labor on what does not satisfy? Listen, listen to me, and eat what is good, and you will delight in the richest of fare."*

Daniel 1:8–16 (NIV) – *"But Daniel resolved not to defile himself with the royal food and wine, and he asked the chief official for permission not to defile himself this way. Now God had caused the official to show favor and compassion to Daniel, but the official told Daniel, 'I am afraid of my lord the king, who has assigned your food and drink. Why should he see you looking worse than the other young men your age? The king would then have my head because of you.'*

Daniel then said to the guard whom the chief official had appointed over Daniel, Hananiah, Mishael and Azariah, 'Please test your servants for ten days: Give us nothing but vegetables to eat and water to drink. Then compare our appearance with that of the young men who eat the royal food, and treat your servants in accordance with what you see.' So he agreed to this and tested them for ten days.

At the end of the ten days they looked healthier and better nourished than any of the young men who ate the royal food. So the guard took away their choice food and the wine they were to drink and gave them vegetables instead."

Luke 12:29–31 (NIV) – *"And do not set your heart on what you will eat or drink; do not worry about it. For the pagan world runs after all such things, and your Father knows that you need them. But seek his kingdom, and these things will be given to you as well."*

Acts 10:10–15 (NIV) – *"He became hungry and wanted something to eat, and while the meal was being prepared, he fell into a trance. He saw heaven opened and something like a large sheet being let down to earth by its four corners. It* *contained all kinds of four-footed animals, as well as reptiles and birds. Then a voice told him, "Get up, Peter. Kill and eat."*

"Surely not, Lord!" Peter replied. "I have never eaten anything impure or unclean."

The voice spoke to him a second time, "Do not call anything impure that God has made clean."

1 Corinthians 10:25-31 (NIV) – *"Eat anything sold in the meat market without raising questions of conscience, for, 'The earth is the Lord's, and everything in it.'*

If an unbeliever invites you to a meal and you want to go, eat whatever is put before you without raising questions of conscience. But if someone says to you, 'This has been offered in sacrifice,' then do not eat it, both for the sake of the one who told you and for the sake of conscience. I am referring to the other person's conscience, not yours. For why is my freedom being judged by another's conscience? If I take part in the meal with thankfulness, why am I denounced because of something I thank God for?

So whether you eat or drink or whatever you do, do it all for the glory of God. Do not cause anyone to stumble, whether Jews, Greeks or the church of God—even as I try to please everyone in every way. For I am not seeking my own good but the good of many, so that they may be saved."

Philippians 3:17-21 (NIV) – *"Join together in following my example, brothers and sisters, and just as you have us as a model, keep your eyes on those who live as we do. For, as I have often told you before and now tell you again even with tears, many live as enemies of the cross of Christ. Their destiny is destruction, their god is their stomach, and their glory is in their shame. Their mind is set on earthly things. But our citizenship is in heaven. And we eagerly await a Savior from there, the Lord Jesus Christ, who, by the power that enables him to bring everything under his control, will* *transform our lowly bodies so that they will be like his glorious body."*

1 Timothy 4:4–5 (NIV) – *"For everything God created is good, and nothing is to be rejected if it is received with thanksgiving, because it is consecrated by the word of God and prayer."*

Exercise and Bodily Stewardship

Proverbs 3:7–8 (NIV) – *"Do not be wise in your own eyes; fear the Lord and shun evil. This will bring health to your body and nourishment to your bones."*

Proverbs 4:20–22 (NIV) – *"My son, pay attention to what I say; turn your ear to my words. Do not let them out of your sight, keep them within your heart; for they are life to those who find them and health to one's whole body."*

Proverbs 14:30 (NIV) – *"A heart at peace gives life to the body, but envy rots the bones."*

Proverbs 17:22 (NIV) – *"A cheerful heart is good medicine, but a crushed spirit dries up the bones."*

1 Corinthians 6:19–20 (NIV) – *"Do you not know that your bodies are temples of the Holy Spirit, who is in you, whom you have received from God? You are not your own; you were bought at a price. Therefore honor God with your bodies."*

1 Corinthians 9:24–27 (NIV) – *"Do you not know that in a race all the runners run, but only one gets the prize? Run in such a way as to get the prize. Everyone who competes in the games goes into strict training. They do it to get a crown that will not last, but we do it to get a crown that will last forever. Therefore I do not run like someone running aimlessly; I do not fight like a boxer beating the air. No, I strike a blow to my body and make it my slave so that after I have preached to others, I myself will not be disqualified for the prize."*

2 Corinthians 7:1 (NIV) – *"Therefore, since we have these promises, dear friends, let us purify ourselves from everything that contaminates body and spirit, perfecting holiness out of reverence for God."*

1 Thessalonians 5:23 (NIV) – *"May God himself, the God of peace, sanctify you through and through. May your whole spirit, soul and body be kept blameless at the coming of our Lord Jesus Christ."*

1 Timothy 4:1-10 (NIV) – *"The Spirit clearly says that in later times some will abandon the faith and follow deceiving spirits and things taught by demons. Such teachings come through hypocritical liars, whose consciences have been seared as with a hot iron. They forbid people to marry and order them to abstain from certain foods, which God created to be received with thanksgiving by those who believe and who know the truth. For everything God created is good, and nothing is to be rejected if it is received with thanksgiving, because it is consecrated by the word of God and prayer.*

If you point these things out to the brothers and sisters, you will be a good minister of Christ Jesus, nourished on the truths of the faith and of the good teaching that you have followed. Have nothing to do with godless myths and old wives' tales; rather, train yourself to be godly. For physical training is of some value, but godliness has value for all things, holding promise for both the present life and the life to come. This is a trustworthy saying that deserves full acceptance. That is why we labor and strive, because we have put our hope in the living God, who is the Savior of all people, and especially of those who believe."

3 John 1:2 (NIV) – *"Dear friend, I pray that you may enjoy good health and that all may go well with you, even as your soul is getting along well."*

Chapter 10: A Traveler's Checklist

Essentials for a Healthy Eating Lifestyle

"Commit to the L*ORD whatever you do, and He will establish your plans."* – Proverbs 16:3 (NIV)

This final chapter brings together the essential food choices and guiding principles of the *Road Map to a Healthy Eating Lifestyle,* as detailed in the other chapters. It is intended as a reference point, not a stand-alone guide, and assumes familiarity with the concepts developed in earlier chapters.

Because metabolisms can vary from individual to individual, some healthy eaters may find that what is a food to eat regularly hinders healthy eating progress. The same may be true with carbohydrates. When the suggested list of food items is not working for you, be sure to experiment with adding and removing items from the list. Also be sure to follow the latest findings on healthy eating and its impact on your metabolism, as research does change over time.

Foods to Eat Regularly

Quality Protein (Base Fuel)
Beef options such as hamburger, steak, and roast; poultry options including chicken breast, thighs, and wings; fish options led by salmon, sardines, trout, and tuna; eggs

prepared whole; and pork cuts such as chops or tenderloin, when minimally processed.

Healthy Fats (Support Fuel)
Natural fats paired with protein, including butter, ghee, beef tallow, and poultry fat; plant-based fats such as olive oil, avocado oil, coconut oil, and whole avocados; olives and olive products without added sugars.

Low-Carbohydrate Vegetables (Supplemental Fuel)
Non-starchy vegetables such as leafy greens, broccoli, cauliflower, zucchini, squash, asparagus, peppers, and cucumbers; root vegetables used selectively, such as sweet potatoes or winter squash.

Dairy (Optional and Selective)
Full-fat options such as butter, heavy cream, and plain full-fat yogurt; cheeses without added starches or sugars.

Beverages
Water as the primary beverage; unsweetened tea; black coffee or coffee with approved fats; broth or bone broth without added sugars or fillers.

Foods That Disrupt Progress

Refined Carbohydrates
Bread, rolls, tortillas, pasta, rice, cereal, crackers, chips, and baked goods.

Sugars and Sweeteners
Table sugar, honey, syrups, agave, fruit juice, sweetened beverages, desserts, and candy; artificial sweeteners that promote cravings or insulin response.

Processed and Ultra-Processed Foods
Packaged meals, boxed mixes, snack foods, fast-food items, and products with long ingredient lists or unrecognizable additives.

Seed and Industrial Oils
Corn oil, soybean oil, canola oil, vegetable oil, sunflower oil, and products primarily made with these oils.

High-Carbohydrate Fruits and Starches
Bananas, grapes, apples, dried fruit, potatoes, corn, and starchy legumes are used as staples rather than exceptions.

Alcohol
Beer, wine, cocktails, and spirits, particularly when combined with carbohydrates or consumed frequently.

Core Principles to Keep in View

1. **Food Quality Comes First**
   Prioritize real, whole foods, organic selections when possible.
2. **Protein Leads Every Meal**
   Begin meals with sufficient protein to support satiety, muscle preservation, and metabolic stability.
3. **Healthy Fats are Paired with Protein**
   Fats support energy and satisfaction when consumed alongside protein, not in isolation.
4. **Carbohydrates are Managed, Not Eliminated**
   Carbohydrates are intentionally chosen, kept low, and balanced with protein to avoid metabolic overload.
5. **Eating Windows Support Metabolic Health**
   Structured eating patterns are tools, not rigid rules, and need to be varied to avoid metabolic predictability.
6. **Consistency Matters More than Perfection**
   Daily adherence to principles outweighs occasional deviations.

7. **Progress is Measured Over Time**
   Focus on trends rather than short-term fluctuations in terms of inches, weight, and energy—consistency matters.

8. **Rest and Recovery are Part of the Journey**
   Sleep and recovery protect metabolic health and support long-term sustainability.

9. **Expect and Plan for Disruptions**
   Travel, holidays, and invitations to eat out happen; returning to the route promptly is more important than avoiding them, as it encourages staying on the journey.

10. **Adaptability Sustains Progress**
    The *Road Map* emphasizes adjustment, awareness, and long-term practice rather than strict adherence to a single pattern.

About the Author

Mark Simpson, Ph.D., brings a practical, personal perspective on healthy living, shaped by his decades-long struggle with weight loss. Rather than proposing quick solutions that rarely lead to long-term success, he emphasizes developing weight loss practices grounded in current research on sound nutrition choices that work with the body's metabolism rather than against it. Sustainable healthy eating, in his view, is best understood as an outcome of choosing to live a healthy lifestyle rather than following a temporary or restrictive eating plan. Following this strategy, he lost 140 pounds over the course of a year.

The *Road Map to a Healthy Eating Lifestyle* reflects the integration of personal experience and professional discipline that characterizes Dr. Simpson's professional work as VP for Academic Services for Rockbridge International Seminary. Written with the structure of an educator and the perspective of a fellow traveler, the book is designed to guide readers through practical choices and steady progress. Dr. Simpson utilizes the metaphor of a *Road Map* as a framework to help readers understand weight loss, the role of metabolism in successful weight loss, and the value of adopting lifelong healthy eating habits.

Made in the USA
Monee, IL
04 November 2026

67383829R00085